W9-AXC-345

The New
Menopause Book

The New Menopause Book

Edited by

Mary Tagliaferri, M.D., L.Ac.,

Isaac Cohen, OMD, L.Ac.,

and Debu Tripathy, M.D.

Foreword by Dean Ornish, M.D.

AVERY
a member of Penguin Group (USA) Inc.
New York

AVERY

Published by the Penguin Group
Penguin Group (USA) Inc., 375 Hudson Street, New York, New York 10014, USA •
Penguin Group (Canada), 90 Eglinton Avenue East, Suite 700, Toronto, Ontario M4P 2Y3, Canada
(a division of Pearson Penguin Canada Inc.) • Penguin Books Ltd, 80 Strand, London WC2R 0RL,
England • Penguin Ireland, 25 St Stephen's Green, Dublin 2, Ireland (a division of Penguin Books Ltd) •
Penguin Group (Australia), 250 Camberwell Road, Camberwell, Victoria 3124, Australia (a division of
Pearson Australia Group Pty Ltd) • Penguin Books India Pvt Ltd, 11 Community Centre, Panchsheel Park,
New Delhi–110 017, India • Penguin Group (NZ), Cnr Airborne and Rosedale Roads, Albany,
Auckland 1310, New Zealand (a division of Pearson New Zealand Ltd) • Penguin Books
(South Africa) (Pty) Ltd, 24 Sturdee Avenue, Rosebank, Johannesburg 2196, South Africa
Penguin Books Ltd, Registered Offices: 80 Strand, London WC2R 0RL, England

Copyright © 2006 by Mary Tagliaferri, Isaac Cohen, and Debu Tripathy
All illustrations are created by Ronit Cohen unless otherwise noted. Copyright © 2006.
All illustrations in chapter 6 were created by Wendy Wray and are reprinted
with permission arranged by Morgan Gaynin, Inc.
Chapter 7 is adapted from *Yoga for Healthy Bones* by Linda Sparrowe. Copyright © 2002 by Linda Sparrowe.
Adapted by arrangement with Shambhala Publications, Inc., Boston, www.shambhala.com.
Photographs in chapter 7 are from *The Woman's Book of Yoga and Health* by Linda Sparrowe, with
sequences by Patricia Walden. Copyright © 2002 by Linda Sparrowe, photographs by David Martinez.
Reprinted with permission arranged by Shambhala Publications, Inc., Boston, www.shambhala.com.

Most Avery books are available at special quantity discounts for bulk purchase for sales promotions, premiums, fund-
raising, and educational needs. Special books or book excerpts also can be created to fit specific needs. For details,
write Penguin Group (USA) Inc. Special Markets, 375 Hudson Street, New York, NY 10014.

Library of Congress Cataloging-in-Publication Data

The new menopause book / edited by Mary Tagliaferri,
Isaac Cohen, Debu Tripathy ; foreword by Dean Ornish.
        p.   cm.
Includes bibliographical references and index.
ISBN 1-58333-242-1
1. Menopause—Popular works.   2. Menopause—Alternative treatment.
    I. Tagliaferri, Mary.   II. Cohen, Isaac.   III. Tripathy, Debu.
    RG186.N47   2006   2005053560
            618.1'75—dc22

Printed in the United States of America
1   3   5   7   9   10   8   6   4   2

Book design by Meighan Cavanaugh

Neither the authors nor the publisher is engaged in rendering professional advice or services to the individual reader.
The ideas, procedures, and suggestions in this book are not intended as a substitute for consulting a physician. All
matters regarding health require medical supervision. Neither the authors nor the publisher shall be liable or responsible for any loss, injury, or damage allegedly arising from any information or suggestion in this book. The opinions
expressed in this book represent the personal views of the authors and not of the publisher.

While the authors have made every effort to provide accurate telephone numbers and Internet addresses at the time
of publication, neither the authors nor the publisher assumes any responsibility for errors, or for changes that occur after publication. Further, the publisher does not have any control over and does not assume any responsibility for author or third-party websites or their content.

Contents

Preface

After I was diagnosed with breast cancer at age thirty, I was fortunate to meet Debu Tripathy and Isaac Cohen, two extraordinary practitioners dedicated to women's health. These men have similar visions about the need for research in the area of complementary and alternative medicine. That was a decade ago, and the three of us have raised millions of dollars in grant money to achieve this goal. When we are not sharing stories about our families and travel, telling jokes, or arguing about politics, we are diligently finding innovative ways to generate data on the role of herbal medicine for menopausal symptoms and breast cancer.

Dr. Debu Tripathy is an accomplished oncologist, recognized for his leading role in the clinical development of the groundbreaking new antibody Herceptin for the treatment of breast cancer. Isaac Cohen is recognized worldwide as one of the leading experts in the application of traditional Chinese medicine for cancer and women's health. My background as a practitioner of traditional Chinese medicine and a physician was ideally suited for our long-term collaboration.

I knew we had a breakthrough in our working relationship when, only one year after our meeting, Debu Tripathy, Isaac Cohen, and I embarked on a fact-finding mission to China. Between meetings with oncologists and acupuncturists, we were in an open-air market, haggling over the price of some silk robes, when an English economics professor asked us the purpose of our trip to China. Debu explained we were researching Chinese medicine, and the man skeptically remarked, "Do you really believe in the concept of qi?" When Debu offered an eloquent and passionate explanation of the traditional Chinese concept of qi, as well as a possible rationale for qi based on molecular and biochemical equilibrium, I almost fainted. It was suddenly clear to me, as I listened to Debu clarify our theories and goals, that we truly had been building bridges between the two medical fields—one that was encrypted in poetic explanations and the other locked in plausible scientific theories.

That was ten years ago. Our collaboration has turned into something much greater than colleagues from different fields working together. We have taught one another to see medicine and healing from many different angles. Whereas Isaac and I once viewed herbs simply as powerful healing tools based soundly on two thousand years of anecdotal evidence, we now know that there also is a biological rationale for their healing effects. This dual understanding—how herbal medicine works according to traditional theories, and how herbs regulate functions of the body according to scientific explanations—has given us the ability to communicate with alternative medical practitioners *and* conventional health-care providers, who commonly practice in isolation of each other. Our ability to speak these two different languages has led us to a new field called *integrative medicine.*

This book is the second collaboration for the three of us. Our first, *Breast Cancer: Beyond Convention,* was a huge success both professionally and personally. We were able to combine our unique experiences working from inside and outside the medical establishment—as well as with patients—to provide women with the most up-to-date information about alternative therapies to treat breast cancer. Feedback on our first book from women with breast cancer has been overwhelmingly positive, and, in general, women feel we tackled the range of treatment issues that they grapple with—but that are often neglected by conventional health-care providers—thoroughly and with sensitivity.

In 2002, shortly after *Breast Cancer: Beyond Convention* was published, we set to work on this follow-up volume, *The New Menopause Book*. Our work with breast cancer survivors (many of whom are thrown into an artificial menopause from chemotherapy and other treatments), had taught us that scientific information about alternatives was desperately needed. Also, menopause was a natural spin-off from our work in the field of breast cancer, because from a biological standpoint, estrogen plays a critical role in the occurrence of breast cancer as well as menopause.

In 2002, the results of the National Institutes of Health (NIH) Women's Health Initiative (WHI) study were published in the *Journal of the American Medical Association* (*JAMA*). We were all floored by the results. The study showed that conventional combined hormone replacement therapy increases a woman's risk of breast cancer, heart attacks, and stroke. Today, there are an estimated 40 million American women in menopause, and roughly 80 percent of them will have hot flashes. Conventional medicine offers very few options to HRT, so it was clear what we needed to do.

We gathered some of the foremost experts in women's health to write this book. One of our goals was to find practitioners who—in addition to being tops in their fields—based the advice and treatment plans they gave menopausal women on strong scientific fact, not simply on hearsay or in-office observation. In *The New Menopause Book*, we assembled a fantastic team of experts who rely on scientific data together with clinical observation when they recommend alternative therapies like herbs and botanicals, bio-identical hormones, yoga and stress management, and vitamin supplements.

The often confusing feelings and experiences you will have during this time may be overwhelming. We hope *The New Menopause Book* will help you find your way through the maze of information about menopause and help you to feel more secure in the treatment choices you make. We are very proud of this book; it is the first of its kind to offer such a wide range of choices for menopausal women. We wish you a full, vibrant, healthy life during menopause and well beyond.

—MARY TAGLIAFERRI, M.D., L.AC.

Foreword

I am genuinely pleased to be writing the foreword to this second important book on women's health issues edited by Mary Tagliaferri, M.D., L.Ac., Isaac Cohen, OMD, L.Ac., and Debu Tripathy, M.D. The first, *Breast Cancer: Beyond Convention,* was hailed as a groundbreaking approach to treating breast cancer. *The New Menopause Book* will surely be the same for the estimated 40 million American women who are in their menopausal transition today.

This book is important *and* timely. Today, the average life expectancy for women in the United States is eighty-two years. And, as Dr. Tagliaferri points out in chapter 2, "Although the life expectancy for women continues to increase, the average age of menopause has not. This means that a majority of women will reach menopause, then live approximately one-third of their lives after this monumental change."

Today millions of women suffer with the unpleasant and sometimes debilitating symptoms of menopause, and many are forced to navigate their treatment options on their own. Conventional doctors typically offer women few treatment options, often giving them only a choice between HRT and no treatment at all.

If you are one of these women who has been struggling with symptoms such as hot flashes and anxiousness and are worried about more long-term issues such as osteoporosis and heart disease, let *The New Menopause Book* be your road map.

I am happy to say that women are turning to alternative and natural treatments as never before to treat their menopausal symptoms. Several recent studies show that four out of five women of menopausal age use dietary supplements and herbal medicine and that the general public makes more visits to complementary and alternative medicine practitioners than to their primary care physicians.

Moreover, recently released results from the National Institutes of Health's (NIH) Women's Health Initiative (WHI) study showed that estrogen-progesterone combination therapies resulted in an increased risk for heart attack, stroke, blood clots, and breast cancer. The study also found that estrogen-only replacement therapy resulted in an increased risk for stroke and blood clots and that there were no benefits for reducing the risks of breast cancer, heart attack, and colorectal cancer. More details about this study and its effects on the medical establishment's treatment of menopausal symptoms can be found in chapter 2.

The results of this study have caused many women who had been taking conventional HRT, or who had been thinking of starting it, to reconsider. This book provides you with the science behind both HRT and the natural alternatives, so that you can make an informed decision about your treatment options.

Each chapter in this book is written by an expert in his or her field, whether traditional Chinese medicine, herbal medicine, naturopathy, or women's health in general. The authors describe the symptoms that you may be experiencing such as hot flashes, memory loss, and depression and how to treat these symptoms with specific therapies and herbal remedies. The authors cite references when available to back up their recommendations with solid scientific research. But most important, these experts share with you the wealth of knowledge they have gained from years of treating women like you. In my mind this is an invaluable service.

The authors emphasize two important points about menopause that are vital: (1) Because no two women experience menopause in the same way, it is crucial to explore a range of therapeutic options; and (2) A healthy diet, moderate exercise, and reducing your stress will improve your health and well-being, making it easier to manage menopausal symptoms.

My work for the past twenty-five years has demonstrated that diet, nutrition, and lifestyle changes can reverse the progression of heart disease, *without* drugs or surgery. Before the results of my research were concluded, there was no scientist who had looked at the effects of a comprehensive, healthy lifestyle program on the underlying causes of heart disease. Recently, I conducted the first randomized controlled trial demonstrating that making sweeping lifestyle changes may also slow the progression of prostate cancer. There is no reason to think these same types of changes wouldn't also have a positive effect on other symptoms and diseases—including menopausal symptoms.

A nutritious diet, regular exercise, giving up smoking (if you smoke), and stress reduction (meditation, visualization, behavioral techniques, etc.) are all part of a way-of-life package that has been proven to benefit health and well-being, and is the foundation of my approach.

This is a good time to begin to think holistically about your health. You will see that your mind plays a large part in regulating body functions, and how well—or, conversely, how badly—your body's systems work has a direct effect on how you feel. Stable, trusting relationships make us more resilient to many types of medical problems. This is something that can be applied to the menopausal transition, too: Gather good friends, loving family, and trusted coworkers around you to spend time together, talk, and connect on a regular basis. You'll soon learn that not only are you not alone but that there are many other women going through similar stresses and life changes. Knowing this and connecting with other women who feel the same way is half the battle when it comes to managing the symptoms of menopause.

To be clear, I am not suggesting that the symptoms of hormonal and other physiological changes that occur during menopause are not real—only that you have a choice about the way you experience them. While the end of menstruation is universal for all women, the subjective experience of it is not. It's clear that biological, nutritional, lifestyle, psychological, and social variables all play a part in the experience of menopause.

My advice to each of you is to look at your life as a whole—mind, body, and spirit—and on a continuum—before, during, and after menopause. With this perspective, you'll be better able to feel in control during the bad times and appreciate the good times. Start with a healthy, low-fat diet, moderate exercise, relaxation techniques, and spend some time with people you love. Make an appointment with your health-care provider (doctor, nurse-practitioner, herbalist, acupuncturist) to discuss your specific health concerns and devise a treatment plan together. And of course, I recommend *The New Menopause Book* as your personal resource to help you make excellent treatment choices.

Take charge of this time of your life. Be good to yourself. Do whatever you can to ease your symptoms. And try to enjoy this time in your life as much as you can. It's going to be a long, wild ride—but it will be more than worth the trip.

—DEAN ORNISH, M.D.
Founder and President, Preventive Medicine Research Institute
Clinical Professor of Medicine,
University of California, San Francisco

The New
Menopause Book

1

Menopause: An Entrance to Your Second Adulthood

Gail Sheehy

Gail Sheehy is the author of twelve books; she is best known for Passages: Predictable Crises of Adult Life *(Bantam Doubleday Publishing Group), which remained on the* New York Times *best-seller list for more than three years and was named by the Library of Congress as one of the ten most influential books of our time. Sheehy has written extensively about the stages of adulthood in a number of best-selling books, including* The Silent Passage: Menopause *(Simon & Schuster),* New Passages: Mapping Your Life Across Time *(Random House), and* Understanding Men's Passages: Discovering the New Map of Men's Lives *(Macmillan Library Reference). Her 1999 biography of Hillary Clinton,* Hillary's Choice, *is currently being made into a television movie, and her most recent book,* Middletown, America: One Town's Passage from Trauma to Hope *(Random House), was published in 2003 to critical acclaim.*

Sheehy has been the recipient of the National Magazine Award, the Washington Journalism Review Award as best magazine writer in America, the Headliner Award from the Association for Women in Communications, and the Anisfield-Wolf Book Award in Race Relations. On six different occasions, she has won the New York Newswomen's Club Front Page Award for distinguished journalism. Sheehy was a founder of the Women's Commission for Refugee Women and Children and is a member of the Women's Forum of New York.

"Please, I don't ever want to get old!"

The image in the mirror was that of a woman probably in her late thirties, attractive enough, but from the shrillness of her plea and the swell of bosom riding above her Wonderbra in the window of a very deep décolletage, she appeared a little desperate. Next to her at the sink in the women's room at the downtown New York café was a woman probably twenty years older. They had been chatting. The older woman was quite a bit rounder and wore far less makeup, but she was obviously comfortable in her own skin. She replied with a lilt of adventurousness in her voice.

"Why not? You'd miss all the fun!"

I chuckled under my breath. I knew exactly what she was talking about. I had just left two handsome men of twenty-five who were trying to flirt with me at the bar—me, a postmenopausal woman more than twice their age. I had stopped into the café after attending a particularly depressing play, alone, on a Saturday night. My husband was three thousand miles away, and I was hungry. There were no tables for a single lady at ten o'clock on a jumping Saturday night, so I took a seat at the end of the bar and pulled out my journal to record my delicious day. I had been entertaining my grandchild. I was deep into the story when the first young man's voice interrupted me. "What are you writing, a book?"

"Maybe," I said. "I like to write."

"Okay, I won't bother you."

But after a while, the second young man tried his approach. "Why don't you write a book about me?"

I looked around the bar. It was chockablock with pretty young women with plunging necklines, apparently unattached. I asked the young men why they were wasting their time talking to me. They gave it some thought. I knew it wasn't my neckline. I was wearing a high-necked black T-shirt. It wasn't my shoes; they were sexy little backless numbers with a tiny heel so I could actually walk in them, but they were hidden under my stool. Finally the taller and handsomer of the two replied.

"You look—interesting."

I continued chatting with the two young men, because, as I told them, I'd met my first husband in the White Horse Tavern.

"Your first?" they asked.

"I'm on my second."

They played along. "Then there's time for one or two more."

"Maybe, but it would be a close call. The current husband and I married after a whirlwind courtship of seventeen years."

They laughed. And then they told me all about themselves, which is what twenty-five-year-old men always do. I listened attentively, which is what twenty-five-year-old women may neglect to do. When I was ready to leave, they wrote their names and numbers in the back of my journal and asked me to call them.

I walked thirty blocks on my backless shoes and never felt an ache in my arches.

I give you this anecdote not to brag (well, a little), but to make the point that a woman is never down for the count—unless she allows herself to grow *un*interested in new life and new people. There are two things you cannot afford to lose if you aspire to feeling ageless: your nerve and your health.

The Gateway to Second Adulthood

Menopause used to tag women with the unflattering label "middle age." But Boomer women simply aren't having middle age. Youthfulness is intrinsic to their identity. And, in fact, American boomers are the beneficiaries of a revolution in the life cycle.

I used to be able to tell a woman's age within two or three years either way. As the author of *Passages,* I had trained my eyes to pigeonhole people as in their Trying Twenties, Turbulent Thirties, Forlorn Forties, Flaming

Fifties, or Serene Sixties. But in the new millennium, I must admit, I often can't tell a fit sexy sixty-five-year-old woman from a careworn fifty-year-old. And it isn't just the "resurfacing" techniques like laser and Botox that are so readily available.

It is because women today can *choose* how to age.

In the space of one short generation the whole shape of the adult life cycle has been fundamentally altered. As I described in my updated book, *New Passages: Mapping Your Life Across Time,* we now have time for not one but two adult lives—before and after menopause. In our First Adulthood we are so busy just getting from A to B to C, we hardly have time to think about what life might be like after we are past worrying about proving ourselves to our parents, getting pregnant, and picking up after children. Today the territory of the fifties, sixties, seventies, and eighties is changing so radically, it opens up a whole "Second Adulthood."

Women now reach the apex of their adult lives at age fifty. It's like climbing to the top of the mountain. Suddenly, we have a breathtaking 360-degree view in all directions. It is possible to appreciate the hills already climbed and the dark valleys left behind. We can discern the pattern of our footsteps. Once a pattern is seen, it can be altered and improved.

Menopause is the gateway to our Second Adulthood. It takes us from the choppy years of family and career-building into the more serene stages, where, buoyed by greater self-knowledge and skill in handling others, a woman can hear her own voice and extend her reach into realms never imagined when she was blindsided by the vanities of youth.

Our Second Adulthood we can custom design. Now is the time to make an alliance with your body and negotiate with your vanity.

The oldest women of the Boomer generation turn fifty-nine in the year 2005. A couple of years ago, the AARP did a poll of its newer members in their fifties—Boomer women—and found they see themselves as in midlife more or less indefinitely until they are over seventy. Asked when they thought they would be old, the majority said not until they are seventy-nine.

And guess what? The fastest-growing age group in America is women over ninety. They just keep piling up at the end! So, we are all pioneers in new passages leading to stages of life that are nothing like the "declining years" our parents or grandparents experienced. That makes it all the more important to ask: How can we best manage the passage through menopause and move on to enjoying our Second Adulthood?

The Truth About Menopause

When *The Silent Passage* was first published in America in 1992, menopause was a taboo subject. Within a year of public and media exposure to the subject, menopausal women themselves recognized they wielded a powerful demographic group—with some 40 million American women entering or beyond menopause by the year 2000. Women editors began featuring it, women legislators demanded research on it, and women patients insisted that their gynecologists become better informed about treating it. Yet even today, menopause remains one of the most confusing passages in a woman's life.

The central myth is that menopause is a time when a woman goes batty for a few years—subject to wild rages and deep depression—and after it she mourns her lost youth and fades into the woodwork. In truth, menopause is the bridge to the most vital and liberated period in a woman's life. But the bridge usually does cross turbulent waters. Hormones have a powerful effect on our physical life and our mood. Many women do experience waves of fatigue and bouts of the blues during the menopausal passage. But that is different from clinical depression. And more important, it is temporary.

The HRT Confusion

It doesn't help that our scientific and medical establishments reverse their "findings" and prescriptive advice roughly every ten years. My generation was herded onto hormone replacement therapy en masse. By the year 2000, six million menopausal women were using HRT to relieve hot flashes and night sweats, mood disturbances, memory problems, and vaginal dryness. We loved the promise that those little pills would keep us young indefinitely, and we felt comforted by the rationale that hormones would protect us against the major killer diseases in older women.

One dynamic entrepreneurial woman told me, when she was forty-five, "I don't want to know when I'm in menopause, because I don't want to think I could ever be that old." When she felt the first faint hot flashes and noticed her periods were irregular, she went straight to the obstetrician-gynecologist who had delivered her children and asked for hormones. The doctor put her on what was then the gold-standard commercial HRT preparation—Prempro. She felt better than she had in years.

But seven years later, in July 2002, the entrepreneur woke up—like Rip Van Winkle—and discovered the world had changed overnight. All prescriptive books written before July 2002 became obsolete. The Women's Health Initiative (WHI)—the first large-scale clinical study of women's health in our nation's history—dropped a bombshell on both the medical community and its menopausal patients.

The usual combined HRT regimen of Premarin and progesterone (combined in the commercial drug Prempro) had been found to fail to protect against the number-one female killer, heart disease, and worse, it actually increased some women's risk for a number of fatal diseases, including heart attack, stroke, blood clots, and invasive breast cancer. Women in the study who were taking Prempro—the same preparation on which the entrepreneur depended—were taken off it, and much of the ten-year study was shut down.

The entrepreneur panicked. Along with legions of other women on hormone replacement, she went off the drug cold turkey. Within a week she was awash in delayed menopausal symptoms and worrying that she might age overnight, Dorian Gray style.

What about the first Boomer women to cross the bridge into the menopausal passage—women who are now between their mid-forties and mid-fifties? Having grown up along with the health and fitness movements and having pioneered the sexual revolution, they already had a healthy skepticism of a medical establishment that had been promoting hormone "replacement" for the last sixty years. But their preference for making the transition naturally comes smack up against the challenge of handling menopausal symptoms while holding down a responsible job and wanting to hold up their sexual desire and desirability.

The Women's Health Initiative study didn't consider them.

"Three weeks after I went off HRT, I felt depressed and foggy," was a common complaint. There are clearly many women who notice a change in sleep, mood, cognitive functioning, and vaginal dryness, all related to their postmenopausal lowered estrogen levels. The debate has become increasingly ideological and polarized.

A woman needs to evaluate her own relative risks for negative effects against the benefits of short-term use of low-dose hormone replacement for symptom management. If you are forty-eight with no history of heart disease or breast cancer in your family, you eat sensibly, exercise, and you're not obese, but perimenopause is causing you misery—menstrual flooding, emotional ups and downs, memory lapses, foggy thinking, and/or lost libido—a few years of hormone therapy may save your marriage or your career. On the other hand, if you are fifty-something and your father had a heart attack or your mother had premenopausal breast cancer, you are in a whole different category.

That is why this book is so vitally important. Women clearly have a crying need for *reliable* alternatives to HRT to help them manage their menopause. I put the emphasis on reliable because, given the anxieties over entering menopause now, when there is no magic elixir, women are likely to fall prey to all sorts of snake oil preparations that promise to relieve their symptoms and keep them young and juicy.

Perimenopause

No matter what generation we belong to, or how much information is available, each woman entering this passage has to reinvent the wheel for herself.

Just about everybody has a preconceived idea of what menopause will be like and when it begins. Women accustomed to catastrophic thinking may worry it will hit them as early as their mid-thirties (very rare). Women who are menophobic may refuse to acknowledge they are in menopause. And some of us are just plain ignorant. The first signs and symptoms usually appear in the mid-to-late forties. This early phase we now know by the name *perimenopause*. The length and impact of perimenopause vary enormously, but it is the most symptomatic phase. I remember it all too well.

I was forty-eight and recently remarried, quietly reading on a snowy Sunday night and playing footsie with my husband, when a little explosion went off in my brain. It felt like a power surge. I looked down at the pages I had just finished reading and my mind was blank. I felt hot, then clammy and cold. I laid down but my heart began racing. For the first time since my earliest menstrual period, I felt profoundly ill at ease within my body.

As more mysterious changes followed over the next few months—sudden energy crashes, bouts of the blues, bloating, headaches, heart palpitations, mind fogs, and, of course, hot flashes—I began to wonder if I was losing it. Not only losing my mind, but losing my usual sexual élan. I felt about as desirous and desirable as a slice of day-old bread that's been reheated in the microwave.

I had no reserves of energy or patience. New York cabdrivers are congenitally abusive, but my husband had to restrain me from engaging in screaming matches with ranting and raving cabbies. "You could wind up shot, or worse, on the front page of the *New York Post*." I wrestled with offbeat health problems I had never encountered before, like allergies, fibroids, and migrainelike headaches (from a progesterone toxicity), and had an uncharacteristic susceptibility to colds and flu.

The sensation was of being *outside* my body but unable to manage it. I kept scolding myself: *What's the matter with you? Why don't you act the way I feel anymore?* The worst part was the fear that this metamorphosis was going to change me into an old woman overnight and I would never be the same me again.

Well, I was right about the last part. I'm not the same "me" as I was in my First Adulthood. But I feel like anything but an old woman, despite the fact that I now have fifteen more years of tread on my wheels. All those mysterious maladies subsided as I went over the hump. I came out the other side feeling stronger and surer than ever, and sexier, because I'm less inhibited. But it didn't happen overnight. And it required a lot of reading and experimentation. What I've learned is each woman is her own clinical trial. Because menopause is as individual as a thumbprint.

Moving from perimenopause into *menopause*—the cessation of menstrual periods—and later settling into the calm of *postmenopause,* is usually a full seven-year transition, like all other major life passages. The reward is release to pursue the passion of your Second Adulthood.

Menopause—The Real Deal

Okay, now you have passed through perimenopause and you are in full-fledged menopause. What does that mean?

Women entering the age of menopause today are likely to be holding down a responsible job and have a child or two still at home. Those in demanding careers usually accelerate their efforts between age forty-five and fifty, which is when a woman or a man either "makes it" into the top ranks or levels off. This acceleration in the workplace happens to coincide, for women, with the body's need to "pause" for menopause. Naturally, this creates a conflict.

The rough part of the transition may be only a matter of months. When and if you are in it, you'll know. Now is the time to make an alliance with your body for the future. You will need to sleep more, because your usual night's sleep may be interrupted by sweats. It helps to eat earlier, which makes your metabolism more efficient.

Take the pause. Even if it means cutting back for a while from your usual pace. Better to leave work a little early and take a good nap before dinner than to go to a business cocktail party and break out in hot flashes that send you to the bar, screaming, "Where is the ice water?"

You may find yourself weepy for no particular reason. Or rather, for a reason so deep in your unconscious, you may not connect it with your mood. You are grieving. This is a loss, an emptying of your magical capacity to give life. But that emptying also frees up enormous energy and allows more singular focus on the things you have always wanted to do.

The singer-songwriter Joni Mitchell took the pause. For more than a year, she declined to make the exhausting performance tours that had been the staple of her career. She retreated into a more private zone and focused on painting, an avocation she has always loved but had little time to pursue. Sleeping whenever she needed to, she often found herself getting up in the middle of the night with a burst of creativity. She described her passage to me in a way I've never forgotten:

"I also went over the hump of the middle-life crazies," she said, smiling at herself. "There is a kind of mourning period for those things you can no longer do. But then something happened of its own accord. You can feel a chemical change in your body, as you go over that hump. You have a greater ability to let go and say, 'I don't want to think about that now,' which is the thing I always admired about men." Once the turmoil was behind her, Joni resumed her performing career and went on to achieve the status of icon while still very much alive and still singing.

Take the Pause

Seek out the women's health center in your area. It's a good place to keep yourself current with both medical and integrative techniques. And if you really want to make an investment in your long-term health and well-being, take one week a year at a health spa. It's an opportunity to slow down and focus on your inner journey, even as you are detoxifying and toning up your outer body. You will also be in the company of other motivated women, some of whom will be older but look better and prompt you to say, "I wonder what she's doing."

My commitment is to spend a week after any book tour at Rancho La Puerta, the original health spa in North America, and still, for my money, the best. I'm always impressed by the many varieties of attractive, energetic, flexible older women there. Even those in their sixties and seventies often look spicy. You can tell by the light behind their eyes and by the purpose and push they apply to walking up Mount Kuchama every morning that they value every moment.

We never lose the need for touching. We are animals, after all, and when did you ever meet a dog or cat who didn't need petting? If touching is not available by a romantic partner, then seek out a massage therapist. It's worth the money. Pets are great touchy-feely companions, and the best ones feel your pain. When you're home alone on a Saturday night, don't drown your hot flashes in drink—which only makes them worse. Just curl up with a good vibrator.

No matter what your current intimate life is like, this is the time to begin cultivating interesting, close, supportive, and optimistic friends, who will be there when and if you find yourself alone. Their own vitality will be infectious. And make sure they're not all in your age group but distributed across the age span.

Begin a program of spiritual rejuvenation. This is the time to do it. Build it into a habit. You can meditate or smoke. You can meditate or drink. You can meditate or fight with your partner and coworkers. This is the most important investment program you can undertake at middle life, and one your broker will not tell you about. In American and most West European societies people are led to believe the spirit is separate from the mind and body. The spirit is an area of growth most of us set aside, half hoping the day will come when some soul-stretching peak experience will lift us out of our ordinary consciousness for a glimpse of the sacred and eternal. But we have to prepare our consciousness for taking such a path. And that requires another level of letting go.

Postmenopausal Zest

Women of fifty today are better able than ever to take advantage of *postmenopausal zest*. That term, coined by the pioneering anthropologist

Margaret Mead, has been affirmed by millions of women who continue to be amazed upon entering a new stage of equilibrium once their periods stop. That point coincides today with manifold opportunities to find and pursue your passion, to assume a position of power or influence, to speak out with a respected voice of maturity, and to initiate action.

In my mid-fifties, I attended a conference at Esalen on The New Older Woman. I was one of the youngest to attend, but once I met our group of accomplished women from age fifty to eighty-plus, my hesitation about including myself evaporated. It is a great idea to seek out models among women ten years older than you are. Find an image that allows you to say, "Mmmm, I could live with that." Such models inspire hope—all is not going to be lost—and with hope you will find the motivation, the support, and the strategies that you need to keep yourself . . . interesting.

But one must keep listening to the body. At the end of the conference, we were treated to an Esalen specialty—an aesthetic massage on a clay table in the open air over the ocean. My masseuse was an Adonis. When he finished and handed me a robe, he stammered. "Can I tell you something?" he asked. I said of course. "Your buttocks are very tight."

Short pause. I replied, "Will you marry me?"

But he wasn't handing me a compliment. As I found out some months later, when I made an unexpected lunge on a wet floor, my buttocks were *too* tight, and they hurt! My body was saying, "Whoa! Take it easy on the running, watch the hills, and how about some serious stretching afterward?"

There is growing evidence that one of the most effective exercise regimens is unbelievably simple, available, and cheap. All it takes is two feet and your motivation to move them down the street or around the park twice a day—for thirty minutes each. It will improve your mood, releasing those delicious endorphins. It will give you a short burst of energy (as your metabolic rate rises). It's relaxing. It clears your head. It kicks your neurotransmitters into action so your thinking processes are enhanced, you become more creative, and you are more likely to hit upon an "Aha!" moment, or at least a solution to the problem that has you all worked up. It also aids in weight control, tones your muscles, and strengthens your bones. And if you stretch afterward, it helps to maintain your flexibility.

Don't assume all the changes you notice are rooted in menopause or hormonal fluctuations. Second Adulthood is not for sissies. We are challenged more than at any time of life. Our parents grow frail and die. Our friends, or we ourselves, may have to battle life-threatening disease. That doesn't mean we have to lose heart. It means we have to learn how to be survivors, not victims. The difference is simple but profound. Victims focus on what they cannot change. Survivors focus on what they can change.

Older women have historically enjoyed high status in other, more traditional parts of the world. Finally, enough American women have broken through the glass ceiling, and now the special privileges that should accompany postmenopausal high status are available to those who assume them.

Finding Your Passion—You're Not Dead Yet

I found my model for postmenopause at Rancho La Puerta. Deborah Szekely was a bride at nineteen and was overshadowed for the next twenty-five years by her dynamic husband, the professor who with Deborah pioneered the health spa concept. It wasn't until she was in her mid-forties that Deborah found out she was smart. Invited to serve on boards of directors of San Diego's cultural institutions, she began showing what she could do and receiving affirmation from her peers. As the first inklings of an independent identity appeared, she was punished for it. Her much older professor husband asked for a divorce.

She took the blow with benign defiance. "If I'd had an easy life, I couldn't be the person I am. I'm a great survivor."

Again, after seven years, her life turned over when her second husband pulled the plug on their marriage. He wanted to retire. Retirement was inconceivable to Deborah. In her early fifties, she felt the surge of postmenopausal zest.

"I've decided I will never marry again," she told me then. "Because I've invested a lot in myself and I want to use it. I realize I don't need a husband. I like the freedom."

But approaching sixty, Deborah was *too* free. Her famous California spa, The Golden Door, had earned the designation of Best Health Spa in the country. The dynamic Deborah Szekely was up against an exquisite dilemma: *What do you do when you've exceeded all your dreams?*

"I wanted something to lose sleep over again," she told me.

That comment distilled much of what is missing in the lives of people in their sixties who are proved successes with their dreams mostly behind them. When we're young, we lose sleep over passing tests, starting our families, the striving to get ahead in our work, lots of things. Deborah hungered to be totally involved and committed again and compelled to get results.

Deborah campaigned to have herself appointed president and CEO of the Inter-American Foundation, a government agency created to support self-help efforts of the poor throughout Latin America and the Caribbean. Over the next half-dozen years she was endlessly shuttling among twenty-six different countries to oversee their "in-country service" offices.

One day I visited Deborah in Georgetown. She was about to turn seventy-two. Her eyes were like beams, and she spoke in staccato bursts. How on earth did she sell the government on hiring a sixty-year-old woman who hadn't been in politics? I asked her.

Frankly, she said, the question had puzzled her, too. Years later she asked the young man who had hired her: "There were others much more qualified for the position, even former ambassadors. Why did you put me on the short list?" He said, "Because you wanted it so much."

Then passion is infectious, I suggested.

"Yes." She smiled. "And passion is the right word. It's the same depth and obsession as the erotic passion when you were deeply in love, when you thought about him every minute. Same as when your children were young and always on your mind. The passion takes you above yourself; you don't stew and fret, because you're so focused. Therefore, I expect my body and my health to support me."

In her seventieth year, Deborah Szekely was diagnosed with breast cancer. Already caught up in the whirlwind of creating her own foundation, she was stopped in her tracks, stunned and angry. After fifty years of being a health-and-fitness guru, how dare her body betray her? But within weeks she returned to her usual positive, proactive approach, went ahead with a pleasure trip to Japan, and flew back a couple of days before her mastectomy. Three days after surgery, she was back to her usual formidable pace. When people asked her about her breast cancer, she said, "I don't have cancer. It's in the Dumpster behind the hospital." Deborah has by now entered her eighties and has one less breast but a brand-new dream. She is going as strong as ever.

The culminating stage of Second Adulthood I call the Age of Integrity. It is primarily a stage of spiritual growth. Instead of trying to maximize our control over our environment—a goal that was perfectly appropriate to the earlier Age of Mastery—now we must cultivate greater appreciation and acceptance of that which we cannot control.

Some of the losses of this stage are inconsolable losses. To accept them without bitterness usually requires making a greater effort to discern the universal intelligence or spiritual force that is operating behind the changes we now notice almost daily. Rather than focus on time running out, it should be a daily exercise in the third age to make the moment count. Each moment is like a snowflake—unique, unspoiled, unrepeatable—and can be appreciated in its surprisingness.

2 Sixty Years of Hormone Replacement Therapy: Where Are We Now?

Mary Tagliaferri, M.D., L.Ac.

Dr. Mary Tagliaferri is an expert in the field of integrative medicine. She is one of a handful of practitioners in the United States trained in both Western and Eastern medicine. Dr. Tagliaferri received her master's degree in Oriental medicine from the American College of Traditional Chinese Medicine in San Francisco, California and her medical degree from the University of California, San Francisco (UCSF). Ten years ago, she was one of the founding members of the university's Carol Franc Buck Breast Care Center Complementary and Alternative Medicine Program. Dr. Tagliaferri has spearheaded clinical research to assess the efficacy of herbal medicine for menopausal symptoms and breast cancer. Currently, she is developing therapeutic drugs derived from traditional Chinese medicine at Bionovo, Inc., a pharmaceutical company she co-founded four years ago. She is the lead editor of Breast Cancer: Beyond Convention *(Atria Press, 2002).*

One of my dearest friends asked me, "Why on earth do we call this transition menopause? Shouldn't we call it menoSTOP? There is no pause. It's not like your period comes back or your skin returns to its wrinkle-free self or your memory and concentration ever become as sharp as they once were. And then there were the hot flashes; I could deal with them. But worse than the hot flashes, even though they came every fifteen minutes, was the rage. That's what worried me the most. When the palms of my hands would tingle, I knew it was going to be a bad day; I was afraid I'd chop someone's head off. So did I consider taking hormone therapy? Of course, and believe me, I didn't give a second thought to breast cancer. I was only worried about getting through the next day."

What Is Menopause?

Menopause is technically one year (twelve months) without a menstrual cycle. The phase before menopause is *perimenopausal* (near), and the phase after menopause is *postmenopausal*. While that sounds clear enough, it's actually the year(s) leading up to menopause when women experience what we commonly think of as menopausal symptoms. The perimenopausal period, sometimes lasting as long as six to eight years, is when hormonal fluctuations are frequent and erratic, menstrual irregularities are de rigueur, and many women feel out of control and confused about what's happening to their bodies.

So what *is* happening?

During the reproductive part of your life, your body works to keep your sex hormones at appropriate levels, depending on where you are in your cycle. For instance, at the beginning of your monthly cycle, estrogen levels are low, which signals the ovaries to start growing follicles and prepare to produce a new egg for ovulation. In the middle of the monthly cycle, both estrogen and progesterone levels spike, and an egg is released by the ovary (called *ovulation*). The increased estrogen also causes your uterine lining to thicken in preparation for implantation of the egg. If the egg is not fertilized, estrogen and progesterone levels drop gradually. This drop in hormones signals the thickened uterine lining to slough off, causing menstrual bleeding and the ovary to start the process over again by starting to grow

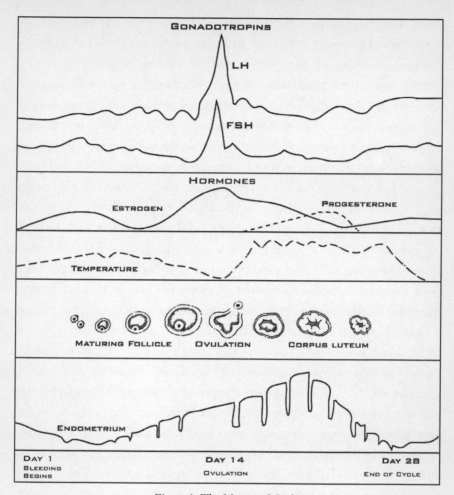

Figure 1: The Menstrual Cycle

more follicles for a new egg and new cycle (see figure 1). Of course, there are women who for various reasons do not have regular cycles.

It has long been believed that a newborn girl has all the ova (eggs) in her ovaries to last her entire reproductive lifetime. However, recent data suggests that eggs continue to be produced in other mammals into adulthood and that this is likely to be true for humans as well. Nonetheless, after a woman reaches about age thirty-five, the number of eggs she has starts to decrease slowly, leading to a drop in estrogen. Normally, this drop would signal the body to prepare another egg, as described above. But without more eggs to work with, the hormonal cycle is eventually disrupted at about age forty-seven, and menopause begins.

While it might make sense to think that *all* the symptoms of perimenopause (hot flashes, irregular menstrual periods, changes in vaginal lubrication, etc.) are the result of a decrease in estrogen levels, recent studies have proven otherwise. In truth, during the perimenopausal period, some of the symptoms (such as breast tenderness, headaches, increased vaginal lubrication) indicate high estrogen levels, and others (night sweats, vaginal dryness, and hot flashes) indicate low estrogen levels. It turns out that what happens during perimenopause is not as simple as a decrease of estrogen that leads to an end of the regular menstrual cycle. At the onset of perimenopause, there is a disruption in your body's normal cycle, and your body reacts to this disruption in a variety of ways. If charted, your hormone levels might look like a mountain range rather than a flat prairie.

Here's an example of what I mean: Let's say your estrogen levels drop. Your body reacts outwardly by producing night sweats and fatigue. But internally, the decreased estrogen is still signaling your body to prepare an egg. While your ovaries may be slower to respond, they are still used to the reproductive cycle you've been living for the past, oh, say, thirty years, so they do respond, eventually. In a last-ditch effort to do what they know, the ovaries may release an abundance of estrogen to get the follicles stimulated and an egg ready. And guess what? This increase in estrogen gives you PMS (premenstrual syndrome) symptoms like breast swelling and tenderness, water retention, bloating, and irritability. Because you still have some eggs available, you will get your period, albeit late, because your ovaries took longer to respond.

The opposite could also happen; that is where your cycle is shortened and you get your period more often. Many women report cycles less than twenty-eight days during perimenopause, sometimes with light menstrual periods presumably caused by anovulation (when no egg is released by the ovary). During perimenopause, some women skip periods completely for a few months, and then go back to a regular twenty-eight-day cycle. The symptoms produced by all these erratic fluctuations may make you feel like a thirteen-year-old girl exhibiting all the moodiness that comes with puberty or a fifty-year-old woman with hot flashes—or both.

Some doctors will try to measure your FSH (follicle-stimulating hormone) levels to determine whether you've begun menopause. This test works well once your period has stopped for a year, as FSH levels do increase at the onset of menopause. However, during perimenopause, you could take this test and have increased, decreased, or the same levels of FSH as during your reproductive years. Some doctors may also suggest testing your salivary estrogen levels; however, there is no conclusive evidence connecting estrogen levels and the start of menopause.

It can be quite confusing. The problem is that it has always been accepted that once a woman begins menopause, her ovaries stop functioning, period. This belief was based on the idea that the ovaries produce eggs and nothing more. We now know ovaries are multitaskers—besides producing eggs, they function as endocrine organs, producing hormones throughout a woman's life. And hormone production doesn't stop with menopause, it just undergoes a transition. Until the transition is over, it's a rocky road as the ovaries adjust to their new, nonreproductive role.

In fact, a woman can become pregnant during perimenopause. You still have eggs, and in most cases those eggs are viable. Fertility is decreased, as there may be some months where you menstruate without ovulating and some months where you miss a period completely. But during those months when you do ovulate, fertilization is indeed possible. So, even though you are being bombarded by your hormones and are sure it is menopause, if you are heterosexually active and do not want to get pregnant, you still have to use contraceptives.

When Does Menopause Begin?

For most women, perimenopause begins between the ages of forty and fifty-eight, although forty-seven is the average age, and full-blown menopause occurs on average at age fifty-one. Unfortunately, there is no definitive factor that determines exactly when your menstrual cycle will become irregular and when the symptoms of menopause will start. Some believe there's a genetic component (i.e., that a woman will begin menopause about the same age as her mother did). However, there are no conclusive studies to prove this theory, merely anecdotal evidence.

One factor that has been proven to affect the onset of menopause is whether a woman has had a hysterectomy. A hysterectomy causes natural menopause to occur two to three years earlier than normal in most women. A hysterectomy is the surgical removal of the uterus, but the ovaries are left intact. Menstrual periods cease when the uterus is removed, because it is the uterine lining that bleeds during your period. Even though after a hysterectomy a woman no longer has menstrual bleeding, if the ovaries are not removed, the rest of the menstrual cycle will continue— producing eggs, estrogen, and progesterone. So, in women who have had a hysterectomy, the timing of menopause may be difficult to judge, as it must be based on various symptoms rather than cessation of bleeding.

Women who smoke cigarettes undergo menopause about two years earlier than nonsmokers. Factors such as number of pregnancies, weight, heart disease, childhood cancer, and age at first period also may influence the age that a woman will become menopausal, but such links are as yet inconclusive. (See the box on page 23 for a description of the types and causes of menopause.)

Symptoms of Perimenopause and Menopause

Each woman's reproductive physiology is unique. Whereas you may have experienced tremendously difficult menstrual cycles—staying in bed with a hot water bottle tucked against your lower abdomen—your best friend may have been one of those lucky women who do not even notice the time of month until a little blood spotted her underwear. Likewise, I've watched many of my friends sail through pregnancy without complaints, while others hug the toilet each morning with unrelenting morning sickness. Even though we all have the same hormones coursing through our bodies, the ways they affect us can be dramatically different. This is

TYPES AND CAUSES OF MENOPAUSE

Menopause can be an event that occurs naturally or a life change that arises out of a medical intervention. In general, the types and causes of menopause can be categorized as follows:

NATURAL MENOPAUSE

Natural menopause is the end of a woman's reproductive years. It is marked by the absence of her menstrual cycle for one full year. This can occur between the ages of forty and fifty-eight, with the average age being fifty-one.

PREMATURE MENOPAUSE

Premature menopause is when a woman's menstrual cycle stops for one full year before age forty. This can occur for a variety of reasons, including genetics, autoimmune processes, or medical interventions such as chemotherapy. Women who go through menopause early have a lower risk of breast and ovarian cancer but are at a greater risk of developing osteoporosis.

MEDICAL OR INDUCED MENOPAUSE

Medical menopause, sometimes called induced menopause, is caused when there is severe damage to the ovaries (such as that caused by chemotherapy used during cancer treatment) or their surgical removal (surgical menopause). More than 50 percent of women on chemotherapy are thrown into a temporary, and sometimes permanent, menopausal state. Older women (over forty-five) are much more likely to experience permanent menopause from chemotherapy treatments than younger women (thirty-five and under). After removal of the ovaries (oophorectomy), the onset of menopause is sudden, and women tend to have fairly severe menopausal symptoms.

why the symptoms women may experience during the years surrounding menopause are many and variable (see the box on page 24 for a list of some of these).

The most common symptom experienced during the menopausal transition is the hot flash. A hot flash is a sensation of overall body heat and facial flushing often accompanied by sweating, heart palpitations,

COMMON SYMPTOMS OF THE PERIMENOPAUSAL AND MENOPAUSAL YEARS

Hot flashes	Anxiety
Irregular menstrual cycles	Urinary frequency
Migraine headaches	Irritability
Heavy vaginal bleeding (perimenopause)	Urinary tract infections
	Heart palpitations
Increased fatigue	Increased itching of vagina
Decreased sexual desire	Forgetfulness
Night sweats	Vaginal dryness
Pain with intercourse	Disturbing lapses of memory
Heat intolerance	Body aches
Weight gain	Emotionally erratic/crying easily
Chills	Loss of self-confidence
Bloating	Easily angered or sudden bursts of rage
Clamminess	Lack of interest in work or hobbies
Increase in facial hair	Lightheadedness, dizziness
Insomnia	Indigestion, gas
Graying hair	Inexplicable feelings of panic
Depression/feeling blue	Disturbing dreams
Thinning scalp hair	Overall sense that you are losing control
Mood swings	Sensory changes in vision, smell, or taste
Urinary incontinence	

and a general feeling of discomfort. Hot flashes usually last between one and five minutes and are often followed by a chill. More than 80 percent of perimenopausal women in the United States, regardless of their socio-economic status, age, race, number of pregnancies, or age at the start of menstrual cycle or menopause, experience hot flashes.[1]

How Women Approach Menopause

Some women look forward to postmenopause as a time when they will no longer have to worry about birth control, and as a time when they no longer have to define themselves by their fertility. Many of the women I have spoken to say they finally feel as though they can relax and enjoy the freedoms afforded to women past childbearing age. Some women express relief that discussions no longer have to revolve around children (or lack of them) and there is more time for pleasurable, intellectual, and professional pursuits. Others feel tremendous loss at the prospect of no longer being fertile, whether or not they were considering having a child or more children.

Our society tends to define women in terms of their motherhood status; therefore it makes sense that many menopausal women feel at loose ends, especially when this is combined with the American preoccupation with youthfulness.

Understanding what is happening to your body can help you feel more in control as the changes begin. Working closely with your medical and/or alternative health provider will help you design a unique plan to suit your changing needs. Staying mentally and physically strong will also serve you well to face the challenges of the menopausal years.

Menopause Is a Modern "Problem"

Menopause is a phase marked by great reproductive and hormonal changes. It is also a new phase in the aging process where women begin to face increased risks from a number of potentially fatal diseases such as heart disease, osteoporosis, breast cancer, stroke, and dementia.

If all this sounds more than a little depressing, think of it this way: menopause and the health risks associated with midlife are simply a by-product of a long life span. At the beginning of the nineteenth century, the life expectancy of a newborn girl was thirty-six and a half years. By the early 1900s, a woman's average life expectancy was forty-five. Today, the average life expectancy for women in the United States is eighty-two years. Although the life expectancy for women continues to increase, the average age of menopause has not. This means that a majority of women will reach menopause, then live approximately one-third of their lives after this monumental change. Currently there are an estimated 40 million women over the age of fifty living in the United States.

Hormone Replacement Therapy (HRT)— The Controversial Menopause Treatment

Hormone replacement therapy (HRT) was introduced in 1942, when the pharmaceutical company Ayerst began marketing the estrogen pill Premarin. (Ayerst was acquired by Wyeth Pharmaceuticals one year later.) By the end of the 1940s, Premarin had been clinically established as a major new drug to combat the symptoms of menopause. (The drug is derived from pregnant mares' urine, which contains high levels of estrogen.)

As time passed, clinical data led physicians to believe that replacing estrogen lost at the time of menopause could prevent or slow down the many signs of aging such as heart disease, osteoporosis, and a decline in cognitive and sexual functioning. This belief was both clinically attractive and biologically believable. The use of HRT became widespread. For sixty years, hormone therapy (the more commonly used terminology in medicine today) was the mainstay of treatment for menopausal symptoms, as well as a preventive treatment for the many chronic diseases associated with aging. It was only in the new millennium that we discovered that many of the studies upon which the medical establishment based its opinions were biased.

In 1986, the Food and Drug Administration (FDA) announced that Premarin and other estrogens were effective not only for treating the symptoms of menopause but also for combating bone loss associated with osteoporosis. As a result, the market for Premarin exploded. At roughly the same time, some studies showed that estrogen therapy benefited the heart as well. A total of forty observational studies conducted over a thirty-year time period suggested that women who took estrogen had a 35 to 50 percent lower risk of coronary heart disease than women who did not use estrogen.[2] At the time, this was a major finding.

An observational study is a study where information about a group of participants is obtained by observing events *without* controlling for particular variables. Observational studies follow participants over time, but there is no drug or therapy intervention. In an observational study, the people involved may have lifestyle practices that are not considered in the analysis, even though they may have a direct effect on the study's outcome. For these reasons, observational studies are generally less reliable than other kinds of studies.

For example, in 1985, the Harvard Nurses' Health study (the largest women's observational study) showed a 50 percent reduction in heart disease among women who took estrogen replacement therapy.[3] It wasn't until seventeen years later that we learned the lower heart disease risk was probably due to the fact that these nurses were healthier in general, exercised more often, ate more nutritious foods and smoked less, rather than the effect of HRT supplements.

HRT AND ENDOMETRIAL CANCER

The first discouraging news about HRT, specifically Premarin, was studies indicating that estrogen-only replacement therapy increased the risk of endometrial cancer. In fact, more than thirty observational studies have demonstrated that the use of estrogen alone for more than ten years increases your risk of endometrial cancer eight to ten times.[4] To eliminate the increased endometrial cancer risk associated with estrogen therapy, progestins were added to HRT. Adding a progestin (a synthetic form of progesterone) to estrogen therapy prescribed to women with a uterus has been proved to remove the increased risk associated with using estrogen alone.

Despite the endometrial cancer risk, hormone therapy looked like a wonder drug, decreasing hot flashes by 80 to 90 percent, thwarting heart disease, and preventing osteoporosis. Because of these celebrated benefits, sales of Wyeth's hormone therapy products, Premarin (estrogen-only) and Prempro (combination estrogen and progestin), were skyrocketing. Annual sales for Premarin reached over a billion dollars by the year 1997.[5] In fact, since the 1990s, the combination hormone therapies using estrogen and progestin have been the most popular treatments for women who have not had a hysterectomy.

In 1995, results became available from an important double-blind study

funded by the National Institutes of Health (NIH) called the Postmenopausal Estrogen Progestin Interventions (PEPI) trial, which confirmed
that hormone therapy has a protective benefit on women's hearts.

In contrast to observational studies, placebo-controlled, double-blind,
randomized trials are the "gold standard" for clinical testing. In this type
of trial, people are included in the study because they meet very specific en-
rollment criteria, the outcomes assessed in the trial are predefined before
the study commences, and participants are randomly assigned to a specific
intervention such as a drug or placebo. Neither the study physician nor the
participant knows to which group she is assigned. Randomization, like
flipping a coin, results in the hormone and placebo groups' being exactly
comparable at the beginning of the trial. For instance, each group will have
just as many women who smoke cigarettes, exercise, and have high cholesterol. This eliminates the major problem with observational studies—
that women who took estrogen were generally healthier to start with.

The PEPI study sought to assess the effect of a placebo and four different hormone therapies (one estrogen-only and three estrogen-plus-
progestin regimens) on a number of key risk factors for heart disease.[6]
There were 875 healthy postmenopausal women aged forty-five to sixty-
four enrolled in the study, who were randomly assigned to one of the five
treatment groups and followed for three years. All four of the hormone
therapy regimens increased HDL, the good cholesterol, and decreased
LDL, the bad cholesterol. Estrogen alone was the most effective therapy
at increasing HDL, but, compared with the other hormone treatments, it
had a significant increase in changes associated with endometrial cancer,
making it a risky therapy for most women, except those who had previously had a hysterectomy.

HRT AND OTHER SERIOUS ILLNESSES

Also in 1995, there were other indications that hormone therapy wasn't
the panacea for all potential complications of menopause. In this year,
a combined analysis of fifty-one studies, including more than 52,000

women, found the risk of breast cancer to be 35 percent greater in women who used hormone therapy for more than five years.[7]

In 2000, a study of more than 46,000 postmenopausal women published in the *Journal of the American Medical Association* (*JAMA*) also found that adding progestins to hormone therapy increased the risk of breast cancer more than with estrogen-only regimens.[8] Furthermore, the addition of progestins blunted the beneficial effect that estrogen-only therapy had on increasing HDL.

The last important study prior to the Women's Health Initiative (the recent groundbreaking study about long-term use of HRT), was the Heart and Estrogen/Progestin Replacement Study (HERS). Since there was already a wealth of observational data supporting the notion that estrogen replacement therapy reduced the risk of heart disease, Wyeth paid millions of dollars to conduct a "gold standard" trial to assess whether hormone therapy in the form of Prempro could prevent a second heart attack in a group of 2,763 women who had already had heart disease.

This was an extremely pivotal trial because no estrogen or estrogen-plus-progestin combination product had been studied in a large, randomized clinical trial, and no form of hormone therapy had received FDA approval for heart disease prevention. Since heart disease is the leading cause of death among women, taking the lives of approximately 500,000 annually, the benefit of a drug that could reduce heart disease among women was enormous. Unfortunately, and to everyone's amazement, HERS had shocking results. When compared with placebo, Prempro led to more heart attacks and deaths in the first year of the study, and with follow-up, there turned out to be no overall cardiovascular benefit.

This roller-coaster history set the stage for the long-awaited results of the Women's Health Initiative, initially published in the summer of 2002.

THE WOMEN'S HEALTH INITIATIVE

The Women's Health Initiative (WHI) was a project funded by the National Institutes of Health (NIH) to determine the effects of postmeno-

pausal hormone therapy on cardiovascular disease, cancer, and osteoporosis. There were two randomized clinical trials: one was designed to
assess the effect of estrogen plus progestin (Prempro) in women with a
uterus, and a second was designed to determine the effect of estrogen-
only (Premarin) in women without a uterus. Premarin and Prempro
were the two chosen therapies because these were the most frequently
prescribed treatments by physicians.

In the estrogen-plus-progestin component of the WHI, there were
16,608 women between the ages of fifty and seventy-nine recruited from
forty different medical centers. This part of the project was a randomized, placebo-controlled, double-blind study of postmenopausal women
comparing the standard dose of Prempro with a placebo. The planned
follow-up time period for each participant was 8.5 years, but the trial was
stopped early because it quickly became apparent that the risks of hormone therapy outweighed the benefits. On average, women were followed for 5.2 years.

The initial study results were published on July 17, 2002, in *JAMA* and
showed that the standard dose of combination hormone therapy caused
an increased risk for coronary heart disease as well as a number of other
potentially fatal diseases including stroke, pulmonary embolism (blood
clots in the lungs), deep venous thrombosis (blood clots in the legs),
breast cancer, and dementia.[9] Moreover, hormone therapy failed to show
any improvement in other quality-of-life measures such as general
health, vitality, mental health, depressive symptoms, or sexual satisfaction.[10] The only upside to Prempro in the study was a decrease in risk for
hip fractures and colon cancer. In the fifty- to fifty-four-year-old women
in the trial, menopause-related sleep disturbances improved with hormone therapy, but there was more vaginal bleeding and breast tenderness. The clinical outcomes associated with Prempro use in the WHI
study are listed in the table on page 31.

Clinical Outcomes per 10,000 Women Treated Each Year from the WHI Study Comparing Prempro with a Placebo

Clinical Outcome	Prempro Group	Placebo Group	Additional Cases per Year per 10,000 Women on Prempro	Relative Risk* for the Outcome If on Prempro
RISKS				
Coronary heart disease	37	30	7 more	29% higher
Stroke	29	21	8 more	41% higher
Pulmonary embolism	16	8	8 more	113% higher
Venous thrombosis	34	16	18 more	11% higher
Invasive breast cancer	38	30	8 more	26% higher
Dementia	45	22	23 more	105% higher
BENEFITS				
Colon cancer	10	16	6 fewer	37% lower
Hip fractures	10	15	5 fewer	34% lower

*Relative risk is the ratio of the incidence of the condition in women on hormone therapy compared with the placebo group.

RESULTS FROM THE ESTROGEN-ONLY TRIAL

While the WHI estrogen-plus-progestin trial was terminated early because of the risks, the estrogen-only trial proceeded under careful scrutiny. This trial included 10,739 postmenopausal women between the ages of fifty and seventy-nine, all of whom had had a prior hysterectomy. Again, researchers were looking at rates of coronary heart disease, cancer, blood clots, osteoporosis, and dementia. But, like the estrogen-plus-progestin part of the study, the estrogen-only study was ultimately stopped early, not because of predefined stopping rules, but because the NIH was concerned about the risk for stroke among the remaining women who were taking estrogen. After an average follow-up of 6.8 years, it was determined that estrogen-only treatment increases the risk of stroke by 39 percent and decreases the risk of hip fractures by 39 percent.[11] (In real numbers, that is 12 additional strokes per 10,000 women and 6 fewer fractures per 10,000 women treated annually.) As was not the case in the estrogen-plus-progestin study, though, the risks for coronary heart disease, breast cancer, and blood clots in the legs and lungs were not increased. In contrast to combination therapy, estrogen-only treatment provided no protective benefit against colon cancer. Among women taking estrogen, there was also a trend for increased dementia.

What the Findings Mean for You

There are a number of important points about the WHI results. First, the average age of the participants in the Women's Health Initiative was approximately sixty-three. However, the perimenopausal period, when women tend to be most symptomatic, starts on average at age forty-seven. Since the absolute risk for many diseases doubles with each decade of life, a woman at age forty-seven who decides to take hormone therapy will have a risk that is *at most* half of what we saw in the WHI trial.[12] For example, in the study, it was found that the relative risk of having a stroke was 41 percent greater for women who were on Prempro. That number sounds shocking, but in absolute terms, the risk is not so dramatic. For every 10,000 women treated each year with the combination therapy in the WHI, there were 8 more cases of stroke than there would have been otherwise.

Now, apply that to a perimenopausal woman who started combination hormone therapy between the ages of forty-seven and fifty and that risk would be reduced by at least half, with the absolute risk being fewer than 4 additional cases of stroke per 10,000 women treated annually. For one year of treatment, this risk is very small, especially if treatment results in the relief of hot flashes, sweats, and insomnia. On the other hand, this small risk is cumulative. For example, if hormone therapy is continued for ten years, the estimated risk for stroke is 40 per 10,000, or 1 in 250 women.

You may also wonder what your risk is of developing any one of the potentially fatal conditions associated with hormone therapy. The investigators from the WHI study calculated the net effect of combination hormone therapy by assuming all of the potentially fatal diseases affected by hormone therapy are weighted equally. They found that combination therapy resulted in 2 serious adverse conditions per 1,000 women treated for one year. The risk is cumulative, so it dramatically increases after five years of treatment to 10 potentially fatal conditions per 1,000 women treated, or 1 in 100. In other words, for a forty-seven- to fifty-year-old woman who wants to take combination hormone therapy for one year, the risk of developing a serious adverse event such as heart disease, stroke, pulmonary embolism, or breast cancer is 1 in 1,000.[13]

Using this information, it's up to you to decide how much of a risk you are willing to take. Are you willing to gamble that you'll be one of the 999 women out of 1,000 each year who have no serious adverse side effects from the treatment? Or are you too nervous about the potential of being the 1 out of 1,000 who develops a serious side effect like heart disease, stroke, or breast cancer to consider taking the hormones? This is something I recommend you discuss with your doctor before you decide about how to manage your menopausal symptoms. And your decision may be based to a greater or lesser degree on how much you are affected by the symptoms of menopause.

Estrogen-only treatment is less risky than the combination therapies (an increased risk of only one serious adverse event—stroke; rather than of four—coronary heart disease, stroke, pulmonary embolism, and breast cancer). This seems to make it a safer drug choice for short-term treatment in low doses. However, if your uterus is still intact, you have to weigh the side effects of vaginal bleeding and greater risk for developing endometrial cancer before you start this treatment regimen.

So, each woman must weigh the risks and benefits of HRT for herself in order to make a good decision about treatment. At the same time, you'll also need to consider your family history and lifestyle choices to determine how likely it is that you will be one of the women who develops a serious illness after taking hormonal supplements.

One important caveat: Whether you read about research studies in the newspapers or hear about them from your physician, there are three questions that you should always keep in mind.

1. Does the population of people included in the study represent my age bracket and medical background?
2. What are the results? (If you don't understand them, have someone qualified explain them to you.)
3. How will the results affect my decision?

Factors That Increase or Decrease Risk of Disease for Women in Estrogen-Plus-Progestin Therapy

DISEASE	FACTORS THAT INCREASE RISK	FACTORS THAT DECREASE RISK
Heart disease	Cigarette smoking High blood pressure High cholesterol Diabetes mellitus Obesity Physical inactivity Family history of early heart disease (before age 55 in men and before age 65 in women)	Regular exercise High HDL and low LDL cholesterol Healthy diet Ideal body mass index* less than 25 (calculated as weight in kilograms/ height^2 in meters)

Disease	Factors That Increase Risk	Factors That Decrease Risk
Stroke	Cigarette smoking High blood pressure High cholesterol Diabetes Obesity Physical inactivity Carotid or other artery disease Atrial fibrillation Family history	Regular exercise High HDL and low LDL cholesterol Healthy diet Ideal body mass index* less than 25 (calculated as weight in kilograms/height^2 in meters)
Breast cancer	Advancing age Starting menstrual cycle younger than age 12 Menopause at age 55 or older No children by birth or first child after age 30 Past breast biopsies with hyperplasia Close relatives with breast or ovarian cancer Genetic risk factors: BRCA1 or BRCA2 genes	Having your first child before age 30 Breast-feeding Regular exercise Avoiding alcohol
Pulmonary embolism	Prior history of blood clots Extensive surgery Marked immobility, before or after a surgical procedure Major orthopedic surgery Fracture of pelvis, femur, or tibia Malignancies Hypercoagulable states	

*Body mass index is a formula used to determine if someone is overweight (BMI > 25–30) or obese (BMI > 30). Normal BMI is 19–25. People with higher BMIs are at higher risk for certain diseases.

As a physician, I'm very frustrated that our current health-care system affords us so little time to address questions like these in sufficient detail with our patients. Still, as a patient, you should be prepared to ask these and other questions of your doctor and demand thoughtful answers.

See the table on pages 34–35 for a list of general factors that would increase or decrease your risk for heart disease, stroke, breast cancer, and pulmonary embolism.

New HRT Recommendations

On the basis of recent research, particularly the WHI study, the FDA has modified its treatment advice for HRT (see the table below). Manufacturers must add warnings about the risks of hormone therapy to their packaging and explicitly state that hormone therapy should not be used to prevent heart disease. Moreover, the FDA now advises women to use estrogens or estrogen-plus-progestin products in the lowest possible doses for the shortest time to reach treatment goals, although it is not

FDA's Approvals and Revised Treatment Advice for Estrogen and Estrogen-Plus-Progestin Before and After the WHI Results		
DISEASE OR INDICATION	APPROVAL PRIOR TO THE WHI	REVISED TREATMENT ADVICE BY FDA SINCE PUBLICATION OF THE WHI RESULTS
Hot flashes	Estrogen and estrogen-plus-progestin treatment is approved for moderate to severe vasomotor symptoms associated with menopause (hot flashes and night sweats).	For hot flashes, estrogen and estrogen-plus-progestin products are the most effective approved therapies.

Disease or Indication	Approval Prior to the WHI	Revised Treatment Advice by FDA Since Publication of the WHI Results
Vulvar and vaginal atrophy (dryness, itching, and burning)	Estrogen and estrogen-plus-progestin treatment should be used for moderate to severe symptoms of vulvar and vaginal atrophy associated with menopause.	For symptoms of vulvar and vaginal atrophy, estrogen and estrogen-plus-progestin products are the most effective approved therapies. When prescribing solely for the treatment of symptoms of vulvar and vaginal atrophy, topical vaginal products should be considered.
Osteoporosis	Estrogen and estrogen-plus-progestin treatment can be used for the prevention of postmenopausal osteoporosis.	When prescribing solely for the prevention of postmenopausal osteoporosis, therapy should be considered only for women at a significant risk of osteoporosis, and non-estrogen medications should be carefully considered.
Heart disease	No approval	Estrogen and estrogen-plus-progestin treatment should not be used to prevent heart disease.

known at which exact dosage the risks of serious side effects are lowered significantly.

One effect of all this new information is that since the publication of the initial WHI results, the sales revenues for Wyeth's Premarin family of products have been on the decline. In light of the new FDA treatment recommendations, Wyeth has received FDA approval for a lower-dose single tablet of Prempro.

The bottom line is that estrogen is the most effective treatment for hot flashes, but using it poses a small risk for serious adverse effects. So if your symptoms are tolerable, it's better not to take any medication. If you have severe hot flashes that don't respond to alternative therapies, you might try a low dose of estrogen. You can increase the dose if you don't obtain adequate relief. Any type of estrogen is effective for hot flashes. You might start with a low dose of estradiol given as a skin patch or gel. While there is no good proof, there are theoretical reasons to believe that applying estradiol via the skin will cause fewer side effects than taking conjugated estrogens orally.

Investigators are currently studying the effects of lower doses of estrogen, and results from those trials will be available soon. Be aware that short-term side effects could occur, like irregular vaginal bleeding or spotting, headaches, nausea, fluid retention, and breast swelling and tenderness. These symptoms are completely normal when taking estrogen supplements and should subside or disappear over time—often in about three months.

Oral Estrogen and Estrogen/Progestin Products

Estrogen Pills	Progestin Pills	Estrogen-plus-Progestin Pills
Premarin: conjugated equine estrogens	Amen: medroxyprogesterone acetate	Premphase: conjugated equine estrogens and medroxyprogesterone acetate
Cenestin: synthetic conjugated estrogens	Cyrin: medroxyprogesterone acetate	Prempro: conjugated equine estrogens and medroxyprogesterone acetate
Estratab: esterified estrogens	Provera: medroxyprogesterone acetate	Femhrt: ethinylestradiol and norethindrone acetate
Menest: esterified estrogens	Micronor: norethindrone	Activella: 17-beta-estradiol and norethindrone acetate

Estrogen Pills	Progestin Pills	Estrogen-plus-Progestin Pills
Ortho-Est: esterified estrogens	Nor-QD: norethindrone	Ortho-Prefest: 17-beta-estradiol and norgestimate
Ogen: estropipate	Aygestin: norethindrone acetate	
Estrace: micronized 17-beta-estradiol	Ovrette: norgestrel	
	Prometrium: progesterone USP	

Gels, Creams, Patches, and Other Products

ESTROGEN PRODUCTS		
Creams	Estrace	micronized 17-beta-estradiol
	Ortho-Dienestrol	dienestrol
	Premarin	conjugated equine estrogens
Vaginal tablet	Vagifem	estradiol hemihydrate
Vaginal ring	Estring	micronized 17-beta-estradiol
Skin patches	Alora	micronized 17-beta-estradiol
	Climara	micronized 17-beta-estradiol
	Esclim	micronized 17-beta-estradiol
	Estraderm	micronized 17-beta-estradiol
	Vivelle	micronized 17-beta-estradiol
	Vivelle-Dot	micronized 17-beta-estradiol

(continued)

Gels, Creams, Patches, and Other Products		
PROGESTIN PRODUCTS		
Vaginal gel	Crinone	Progesterone
ESTROGEN-PLUS-PROGESTIN PRODUCTS		
Skin patch	CombiPatch	17-beta-estradiol and norethindrone acetate
	Ortho-Prefest	17-beta-estradiol and norgestimate

If you are considering treatment primarily for osteoporosis, there are a number of newer drugs available that do not have the same adverse effects as estrogens. (To read more about available treatments for osteoporosis, see chapter 6.)

See the tables on pages 38–40 for a list of all hormone therapies approved by the FDA.

Other Drugs Proven to Treat Hot Flashes

Hormone therapy is generally not prescribed for women with a history of breast cancer, because there is an increased risk for breast cancer with HRT.[14] Many women, especially those with a history of breast cancer, are turning to alternatives to alleviate their hot flashes and night sweats.

There are a few nonhormonal prescription drugs (like antidepressants) that have undergone testing in clinical trials as a treatment in reducing hot flashes. These drugs have mostly been tested on women who have a history of breast cancer—except for Paxil and Neurontin.

The table on pages 41–42 lists the nonhormonal pharmaceutical drugs that have been evaluated in clinical studies for their ability to reduce hot flashes. The drugs found to be most effective in alleviating hot flashes were the newer antidepressants: Effexor and Paxil. Although

Nonhormonal Pharmaceutical Agents for Hot Flashes

Drug Classification	Drug Name	Clinical Effect on Hot Flash Score or Frequency[15]	Commonly Reported Side Effects

Antidepressant	Venlafaxine (Effexor)	Hot Flash Score
		
		Placebo:
		    27% reduction
		
		37.5 mg/day:
		    37% reduction
		
		75 mg/day and 150 mg/day:
		    61% reduction
			Mouth dryness
			Nausea
			Constipation
			Anxiety
			Sexual disturbances
			Dizziness
			Somnolence

Antidepressant	Fluoxetine (Prozac)	Hot Flash Score
		
		Placebo:
		    36% reduction
		
		20 mg/day:
		    50% reduction
			Mouth dryness
			Nausea
			Constipation
			Anxiety
			Sexual disturbances
			Somnolence

Antidepressant	Paroxetine (Paxil)	Hot Flash Score
		
		Placebo:
		    27% reduction
		
		12.5 mg/day:
		    62.2% reduction
		
		25 mg/day:
		    64.6% reduction
			Mouth dryness
			Nausea
			Constipation
			Anxiety
			Sexual disturbances
			Dizziness
			Somnolence

Anticonvulsant	Gabapentin (Neurontin)	Hot Flash Score
		
		Placebo:
		    31% reduction
		
		900 mg/day:
		    54% reduction
			Somnolence
			Dizziness
			Headaches
			Tremors

(continued)

Drug Classification	Drug Name	Clinical Effect on Hot Flash Score or Frequency[15]	Side Effects

Antihypertensive agent	Clonidine (transdermal patch)	Hot Flash Frequency
		
		Placebo:
		  27% reduction
		
		0.1 mg/day:
		  44% reduction
			Mouth dryness
			
			Constipation
			
			Drowsiness
			
			Potential for low blood pressure

Antihypertensive agent	Clonidine (oral)	Hot Flash Frequency
		
		Placebo:
		  24% reduction
		
		0.1 mg/day
		  38% reduction
			Mouth dryness
			
			Constipation
			
			Drowsiness
			
			Potential for low blood pressure

these antidepressants are effective at reducing both the number of hot flashes experienced each day and their severity, they can cause a number of side effects. The most common ones are nausea, sleepiness, dizziness, anxiety, dry mouth, constipation, and sexual problems.

Tips for Easing Menopausal Symptoms on Your Own

Throughout the rest of this book, you will learn about alternative ways to treat your menopausal symptoms. Besides using HRT, many women have had success in managing menopausal symptoms by making nutrition and lifestyle changes. I would like to conclude this chapter with a few tips that I have received from patients throughout my years of treating menopause. Here are a few simple suggestions you can try before taking the HRT plunge:

- Dress in layers so you can easily remove clothing when you feel a hot flash coming on.
- Monitor the events that trigger your hot flashes, then try to avoid them. Triggers could include caffeine, hot drinks, alcohol, sugar, hot weather, spicy foods, tobacco, hot tubs and saunas, physical and emotional stress, heated arguments.
- Exercise more—at least thirty minutes five days a week.
- If you smoke tobacco, quit.
- Consider relaxation techniques such as breathing exercises, meditation, yoga, and guided imagery.
- Drink a glass of cold water or juice at the onset of a hot flash.
- Use light cotton sheets and keep your bedroom cool at night.
- Find a relaxing place to sit out your hot flash without interruptions.
- Try to maintain your sense of humor.

We know that no two women experience menopause exactly alike. I tell women that menopause is one condition with at least forty million ways to experience it. This is precisely why you need to individualize your approach for coping with this life transition. In *The New Menopause Book,* you'll find the resources to do just that. Use the following chapters as a guide and allow the leading experts to navigate you through this passage gracefully.

3 Herbal Therapies:
East Meets West

*Amanda McQuade Crawford, B.A.,
MNIMH, Dip. Phyto*

Amanda McQuade Crawford is an internationally recognized expert on integrated health and plant medicine. Amanda lectures to medical doctors and pharmacists on herbal medicine. After four years at the College of Herbal Medicine in England, she graduated with a diploma in phytotherapy. She is also a member of the National Institute of Medical Herbalists (NIMH) and a founding member of the American Herbalists Guild, and has served on several review committees, including those of the American Herbal Pharmacopoeia. A lecturer for the distance-learning International College of Herbal Medicine, Crawford has also published two popular books on women's health, The Herbal Menopause Book *and* Herbal Remedies for Women. *After many years in private practice in Beverly Hills and Ojai, California, she has taken a position at the Canterbury College of Natural Medicine in New Zealand.*

The news about the risks of hormone therapy has resulted in a great deal of interest in alternative methods to treat menopausal symptoms such as hot flashes, vaginal dryness, irritability, depression, and menopause-related conditions such as osteoporosis.

The idea that certain herbs might reduce hot flashes and treat other menopausal symptoms and conditions should not be shocking, since much of our modern pharmacopoeia is based on herbal compounds. For example, the root of the wild Mexican yam has been used as a progesterone source for the birth control pill. Many women are turning to herbs and natural supplements to relieve menopausal symptoms and fight certain diseases because conventional medicine has not come up with treatment options other than HRT.

It is generally known that certain plant compounds can produce similar effects as estrogen and progesterone on humans. However, most herbal formulas on the market for women's menopausal health take the shotgun approach, with too many herbs and not enough of each to be very effective. Some manufacturers just throw together the best known "female" herbs with no practical knowledge about herbs and how they work. In this chapter, I offer you a firsthand look at herbal medicine in the treatment of menopausal symptoms. I explain what herbs are and how to take them, and then I include herbs and their recommended doses and herbal combination formulas that I use in my practice to treat women. The herbs I recommend here include those that reduce stress and the symptoms of stress such as anxiety and depression as well as hot flashes, night sweats, insomnia, and vaginal dryness.

What Is an Herb?

For the purposes of this book, an herb (also called a botanical) is a plant or plant part used for its medicinal or therapeutic properties. Herbalists may use any part of the plant—flower, leaf, bark, berry, fruit, seed, root, even seaweed, mushroom, and moss. Herbal supplements are dietary supplements that contain herbs, singly or in mixtures. Herbs are identified by their common name and/or by their Latin (scientific) name, which is made up of the genus and species names of the plant; for example, Saint-John's-wort is also *Hypericum perforatum*.

Many herbs have a long history of use, and many of the claims made about their healing properties are anecdotal, which is not to say they are not effective. However, it is important to note that many herbs have not been well studied, especially in the United States. In general, herbal products on the market are not approved by the FDA for specific uses and are not subject to the same regulatory standards as drugs, which means that the quality and quantity of the active ingredient can vary wildly. So be sure to look for a product with a standardized amount of the active ingredient.

Remember, just because herbs are "natural" doesn't mean they are benign; herbal therapies can be potent and can act in the same way as drugs. If not taken properly or if taken in excessive amounts, herbs can cause medical problems, and some herbs are known to have negative interactions with some prescription and over-the-counter medications. For these reasons, it is best to work with a qualified herbalist and your medical provider to find the best herbal form, combinations, dosages, and brands.

An herbalist is a person trained in the use of medicinal plants, either through a recognized training program or by apprenticing with an experienced herbalist. For more information or a list of herbalists in your area, you can contact the American Herbalists Guild (www.american herbalistsguild.com).

In recent years there has been increasing scientific study of herbs for a variety of illnesses and ailments—among these are symptoms of menopause, such as hot flashes, insomnia, vaginal dryness, depression, and anxiety. And there have been some very encouraging results.

This chapter focuses primarily on Western herbs, although it does include a few herbs from other traditions such as Chinese medicine because they are routinely prescribed by herbalists in the West.

Andrea's Story

Andrea simply fell apart at fifty-two years of age. She forgot things, slept only a few hours a night, and then couldn't get out of bed in the morning. She had no interest in exercise and gained twenty pounds in one year. She was depressed, sweated profusely—soaking her sheets—at night, and was constantly angry at herself and everyone around her. Once an artist with a colorful, vibrant life, Andrea was unable to concentrate on her painting, and she withdrew from her once large circle of friends.

Andrea's depression, along with the immune system and hormonal changes she was experiencing, were textbook menopausal symptoms. I suggested she take a formula that included Saint-John's-wort (*Hypericum perforatum*), an herb known for treating mild to moderate depression. This herb has a long-standing use in herbal medicine: improving the function of nerve tissue after chronic stress. It also increases the effectiveness of remedies for hot flashes and other menopausal symptoms. Her formula also contained bacopa or brahmi (*Bacopa monniera*), an Ayurvedic herb known for improving mental performance and memory (Ayurvedic medicine is an ancient Indian holistic approach to health and healing); wu wei zi (*Schizandra chinensis*), a Chinese herb (usually prescribed for liver detoxification) to help with hot flashes and night sweats; and Siberian ginseng to help improve the functioning of her adrenal glands and reduce the symptoms resulting from stress. The adrenal glands help us adapt to stress, and herbs that support these glands can ease many symptoms that might otherwise require large amounts of herbs to reduce each separate symptom, such as sleeplessness, poor memory, mood changes, and hot flashes. Last, I recommended rosemary oil, which acts as an antioxidant and helps the body absorb the herbs and dietary nutrients.

ANDREA'S FORMULA

1 g Saint-John's-wort
650 mg bacopa
650 mg wu wei zi
500 mg Siberian ginseng
10 mg rosemary oil

In addition to the herbs, Andrea needed to make some changes to her diet. I recommended that she emphasize lean proteins, healthy oils, and complex carbohydrates—grains, fruits, and vegetables.

Within three weeks, Andrea was sleeping through the night, five nights out of seven, for the first time in a year. Her memory improved so that she remembered to take her herbs every day, and the once self-professed "junk-food junky" began eating nutritious meals rich in proteins and vegetables with small amounts of complex carbohydrates. Soon Andrea admitted she was actually craving fiber-rich fruits and vegetables. She liked how she felt, and she lost five pounds in three weeks. The goal was for Andrea to lose one to two pounds a week until she reached her goal.

After three more weeks, Andrea's depression was dramatically improved but not resolved. Then, a family crisis intervened and she was back in the throes of depression. I recommended valerian, to be taken in soft-gel capsule form—five pills (250 mg each) at a time for two nights—to help her sleep and reduce her night sweats. She was not groggy in the morning, and Andrea was amazed at how quickly she rebounded.

After Andrea had been on the Saint-John's-wort and bacopa for four months, I reduced her dose to one tablet twice a day for each herb for another three months. Andrea was able to work again; she began a new art project, which was both demanding and rewarding. And despite Andrea's hectic ten-week work schedule, her menopausal depression and memory lapses did not return. Andrea told me that she felt revitalized and self-possessed.

After three more months, I lowered Andrea's formula to a maintenance dose consisting of one tablet of bacopa Monday, Wednesday, and Friday, and one tablet of Saint-John's-wort Tuesday, Thursday, and Saturday. She takes valerian only during hot summer nights.

How to Take Herbs

Herbs come in many forms: fresh or dried; liquid or solid extract; and tablet, capsule, powder, and tea bags. But how does one take them? Brewed in a pot of tea? Eaten as a leaf at the new moon? Or swallowed as a tablet out of a bottle of herbs with a bar code?

Which form you choose may depend on personal preference or may be based on the specific knowledge of your herbalist. Traditional medical practitioners from India to the Amazon often use dry or powder herbs because they are easier to mix, ingest, or store until needed. This is what is meant by the term *crude herb. Liquid preparations* of herbs are widely used because they are better absorbed than many commercial tablets or capsules. Using liquid extracts of individual herbs also gives the herbalist or the consumer more flexibility as to dose and herbal combinations.

TAKING HERBS AS TEA

The simplest liquid extract is a cup of herb tea. Two types of tea are commonly used: *infusions* and *decoctions.* An infusion is a cup of tea in which lighter plant parts (dried leaves, flowers) are infused, or steeped, in water that has been boiled. Steeping time varies from five to twenty minutes, averaging ten minutes for most commonly used teas. A tea infusion can be made in beverage strength (1 teaspoon of dried herb per 1 cup of water) or the standard therapeutic strength (1 ounce of dried herb per 2 cups of water). The adult dose is ½ cup four times a day or 1 cup twice a day.

A decoction is a cup of tea in which the denser parts of the plants (bark, root, berries, seeds) are simmered or concentrated in water on a low heat. The amount of tea used is similar to infusions—1 teaspoon per 1 cup up to 1 ounce per 2 cups. The tea is usually covered and simmered for five to twenty minutes. The dose is ½ cup two to four times a day. Decoctions often taste stronger than infusions.

If a formula includes both flowers and roots as ingredients, an easy, one-pot, two-step process will yield the best results. Pour 4 cups of cold water in a saucepan containing 1 ounce total of the specified roots, barks, or berries; bring to a simmer, covered, for fifteen minutes. Turn off the heat. Into the same pot add 1 ounce of the specified amounts of leaves and flowers; re-cover for another ten to fifteen minutes. Strain the tea and drink 1 cup three to four times a day.

TINCTURES AND EXTRACTS

Not all medicinal compounds in plants, such as resins from myrrh (*Commiphora molmol*), extract well in a cup of tea. In such cases, liquids other than water are often used to produce extracts or tinctures, both of which are more concentrated than tea.

A *tincture* is an extract of one herb using a mixture of water and alcohol. In retail and professional practice, the alcohol used is medicinal grade ethyl alcohol. This water-alcohol liquid is mixed with an herb until all the properties of the herb are dissolved into the liquid—usually in about fourteen days. The stems, flowers, and pieces of herb are separated from the liquid and discarded. (Separate herb tinctures can also be combined to make a specific formula.)

This process removes the medicinal compounds from herbs more fully than brewing a tea, which means a tincture is stronger and has more healing potential. A good example of an herb whose healing properties are magnified by taking it in the form of a tincture is black cohosh root (*Cimicifuga racemosa*), which is recommended for hot flashes and other symptoms of menopause. Many herbalists prefer tinctures because the water-alcohol extraction method does not require that the liquid be heated, which protects heat-sensitive oils or other plant parts from damage. Also, tinctures have a longer shelf life than dried herb or brewed tea. Properly stored herb tinctures (such as in dark glass bottles) can retain their potency for one to several years. Expiration dates are provided on wholesale and retail tincture labels. Labels also have ratios, which tell how strong or weak a tincture is. For example, 1 teaspoon of 1:5 tincture is roughly equivalent in strength to 1 gram of an herb, whether taken directly or extracted in one 8-ounce cup of herb tea. When tinctures are stronger than 1:2, they are called extracts.

Commercially, the word *extract* has been used as an umbrella term for any herb product that is not eaten fresh out of the garden. This causes a lot of confusion among consumers as well as the regulatory authority. To make sure you are getting the best herbs, look for herbs from companies whose labels include the scientific names of ingredients, exactly how much of each herb is present in the formula, and a customer-service website address or toll-free phone number. Many of the better companies also are voluntary members of the American Herbal Product Association, a group focused on quality control.

An *extract* is best described simply as a preparation that is quantifiably more concentrated than a tincture. An extract is usually made in the same way as a tincture. Extracts can also be made by percolating the herb (draining or seeping through a filter) using cold solvents (water, alcohol, or other), though in some cases heat may also be used.

An extract may be taken as a liquid or processed into semisolid or powdered extracts (that are stronger than a tincture), tea, dried herb in a capsule, or ground herb in a tablet.

GLYCERIDES

Glycerides (also glycerites) are tinctures made from herbs with glycerine, a by-product of plant oils used in manufacturing. The use of vegetable glycerine is almost as efficient as alcohol for extracting the medicinal properties from plants. It also tastes better—sweet, although it is not a sugar. Typically, the adult dose is the same as for alcohol-based tinctures: 1 teaspoon one to three times a day. Each teaspoon is equivalent to 5 ml, and 6 teaspoons make 1 ounce. Children's doses are often determined by weight rather than age but may safely be estimated at half an adult dose. Excessive use of herbs with glycerine (more than one ounce a day for adults) may cause loose stools or changes in blood sugar in insulin-dependent diabetics.

HERBAL TABLETS

Tablets are a convenient way to take herbs and to avoid the bitter taste of teas and tinctures. However, with tablets, there is a chance that the herbs will pass partially undigested through the digestive system, which makes them less reliable. Another disadvantage to tablets is that herb quality is not always guaranteed (tablets are notorious for being less effective, possibly due to quality issues or absorption problems). There is no way to tell if, for example, coated Saint-John's-wort tablets or pills have the right herb or strength to have an effect, so you must rely on the manufacturer. And preparing tablets for maximum reliability is expensive, and thus cuts into a manufacturer's profits. Most important, tablets that include a combination of herbs may not suit every person. So-called kitchen-sink tablets with a variety of herbs, each in small amounts, may target a set of symptoms, but the user may not have all of the symptoms.

HERBAL CAPSULES

Capsules containing dried, ground herbs are arguably more convenient than tinctures and extracts, and some people find capsules easier to digest than tablets. However, because herbs are so dense in this form, you would have to take a large number of capsules to receive the appropriate medicinal effect. For example, even large capsules contain only 300 to 650 mg of powdered herb, and a standard adult dose for common herbs may easily range from 2,000 to 4,000 mg. This means that to achieve the proper dose, you might have to take as many as twelve capsules. Fortunately, concentrated extracts are now available in capsule form to reduce the number of capsules a person must take for best results.

Below is the story of a patient of mine (her name has been changed) who began having symptoms of menopause in her early forties.

Connie's Story

A forty-three-year-old medical writer, Connie is in early perimenopause. She complains that she is depressed, anxious, and has severe PMS two weeks before her period, with anxiety for one week afterward. Her PMS symptoms include mood swings, skin blemishes, hair loss, blood-sugar problems, weight gain, disturbed sleep, and lack of mental clarity. Her period is still regular, coming every twenty-eight days. Connie supports herself and her husband, who is out of work; they have no children by choice. Connie is afraid of menopause because her mother had a nervous breakdown at forty-five, when she began menopause.

Connie's doctor recommended hormone replacement, which she decided against after reviewing the literature. She tried a natural wild yam cream for three months, which made her skin break out severely, and it did not help her depression, anxiety, or related problems. She was prescribed Zoloft two years ago, which helped her anxiety, but she has felt tired and less mentally clear since she started taking it.

Connie decided to go off Zoloft and began self-treating with herbs (Saint-John's-wort, kava, and several others), but the anxiety returned. Because she was taking so many different herbs, but each at a relatively low dose, the herbs were not having the medicinal effect they were supposed to. When Connie came to see me and told me her medical history, I prescribed two herbal formulas (herb extracts are 1:5 unless noted otherwise):

HERBAL FORMULA #1

6 ounces dong quai (1:2)
3 ounces ginkgo

3 ounces kava
3 ounces Saint-John's-wort (1:2)
16 ounces fennel (1:2)

I recommended that Connie take 1 teaspoon (5 ml) diluted in 1 cup of water (8 ounces) twice a day before meals.

HERBAL FORMULA #2

3½ ounces dandelion root
2 ounces passionflower
2 ounces anemone (1:2)
8 ounces skullcap (1:2)

I recommended that Connie take 1 to 2 teaspoons at bedtime as needed.

In five weeks, Connie reported feeling great. Her digestion was improved; her immune system was strong—no flu or colds; and she was having regular bowel movements and normal urination. We substituted chamomile tea for the herbal formula used at bedtime, to be followed with ½ to 1 teaspoon of tincture only as needed.

After five months on the formulas, her PMS was gone; she's had one bout of flu, but no anxiety and only slight mood swings; her skin was vastly improved. Connie's hair was growing back, she had lost twenty-two pounds, and her blood sugar, energy level, daytime concentration, and sleep patterns were all back to normal. She still took half a Zoloft (25 mg) every day and was ready to drop it to a quarter dose. Our plan was to maintain this until after the next period and then start to wean her off the Zoloft altogether.

After one year of herbal therapy, Connie, now forty-four, was off Zoloft, felt "brighter," and looked forward to menopause as a positive change. The last time we spoke, Connie had decided on a career change: she'd registered at a local college to study integrative medicine.

Herbs for Stress Reduction

The adrenal glands secrete hormones that help you cope with daily stress in healthy ways. However, stress and the way you handle stress as well as environmental and dietary factors can affect the efficiency of your adrenal glands. If your adrenal glands are depleted, you are much more likely to suffer from fatigue and menopausal symptoms. A woman who enters perimenopause with impaired adrenal function is more likely to suffer more extreme symptoms. Signs that your adrenals are on overload:

- You awaken feeling groggy and have difficulty dragging yourself out of bed.
- You need a cup or two of coffee or tea to get going in the morning.
- You crave sugar and caffeine during the day, especially in the late morning or afternoon, and are tired if you don't have them.
- You are exhausted at night but have trouble falling asleep and feel anxious.
- You have lost all interest in sex.

Severe adrenal deficiency requires careful medical evaluation and perhaps replacement therapy. However, for cases of less severe adrenal deficiency, there are less drastic methods for recharging your adrenal glands. The first step to improving your adrenal health, of course, is to identify and reduce stress in your life. Maintaining a healthy diet and taking a multivitamin will also help increase adrenal functioning. There are also a variety of herbs that can be used to boost adrenal functions. Below are some of the herbs that I recommend in my practice for stress reduction and adrenal gland health.

ASHWAGHANDA

Ashwaghanda (*Withania somniferum*) is also known by the name winter cherry and belongs to the pepper family. Ashwaghanda is an important

herb in Ayurvedic medicine. Practitioners of natural and herbal medicine who treat women for hot flashes, anxiety, depression, and loss of
cognitive functions—menopausal symptoms that are thought to be associated with the decline of estrogen—often relate these symptoms to a reduced ability to respond to stress. Therefore, many herbalists recommend
ashwaghanda to increase the body's ability to withstand stress and improve physical energy and overall health. It may also strengthen the
immune system.

Ashwaghanda can be taken as a tea or in tincture form. (There are
also delicious-tasting coffee substitutes on the market that contain ashwaghanda. Follow the directions on the label.)

> Tea: 1 cup of tea one to three times a day
> Tincture: 1 to 3 teaspoons in 8 ounces of water per day, or in
> combination with other herbs

GINSENG

Ginseng, either Asian ginseng (*Panax ginseng*) or American ginseng
(*Panax quinquefolium*), is native to China, Russia, North Korea, Japan,
and some areas of North America. It was first cultivated in the United
States in the late 1800s. Ginseng has become a darling of herbal medicine
and as a result has been burdened with many false advertising claims.
However, some clinical trials show ginseng can aid performance under
stress, cardiovascular health (especially in the middle-aged and elderly),
blood-sugar balance, and mental function.

The main active ingredients of ginseng are the more than twenty-five
saponin triterpenoid glycosides called ginsenosides. These steroidlike
ingredients enable ginseng to balance and counter the effects of stress.
However, because it is a stronger herb than ashwaghanda for reducing
the effects of stress on the body, ginseng is not recommended for
all menopausal women. It works best for women who are exhausted
and have severe hot flashes and/or cardiovascular weakness such as

low blood pressure due to a weak heart, arteriosclerosis, or poor circulation.

For women suffering from menopause-related stress, ginseng may work in the short term by improving stamina and resistance to stress. Over the long term it improves degenerative conditions associated with aging such as risk of heart disease. Ginseng also can blunt the effects of a wide range of physical, chemical, and biological stressors on the body, including radiation.

The best results come when the herb is taken for six weeks or longer.[1] Ginseng is widely used in the United States to improve overall energy and vitality, particularly during times of fatigue or stress; boost energy levels; enhance memory; and stimulate the immune system. Several studies confirm its reputation for improving mental and physical performance, from carbohydrate metabolism to improved memory.[2]

Ginseng apparently affects people differently; for example, it has an estrogenic effect for women when estrogen is low or absent, but in men who do not need much estrogen it increases testosterone and promotes sperm health.

If you try ginseng and it disagrees with you, you will know within one to two days. In some people it may cause headaches, heart palpitations, insomnia, or itchy skin. If you experience any of these symptoms, stop taking the herb and your symptoms should go away immediately. It is not recommended for people with acute asthma, high blood pressure, and, in some cases, insomnia. Ginseng should not be taken with hormone therapy, stimulants (caffeine, amphetamines), blood thinners (warfarin), and monoamine oxidase inhibitors (MAOIs), a class of antidepressant drugs.

Ginseng has very low toxicity, but, as with all herbs, you should practice caution when taking it. The recommended dose is $\frac{1}{2}$ to 3 grams per day. Small women or women who are sensitive to herbs or drugs should take the minimum dose; others can slowly increase the dose to the maximum over a period of weeks as their bodies adjust to the stimulating effects of ginseng. Tinctures are given in the dosage range of 1 to 6 ml per day. Ginseng is best taken early in the day to prevent sleep problems, whether on its own in the above dosage range or in a combination of herbs. The following tincture formula is a good one for treating menopausal symptoms related to stress (this formula will last about two weeks):

1 ounce ginseng (Radix panacis ginseng)
2 ounces hawthorn (Crataegus monogyna)
1 ounce dandelion leaf (Taraxacum officinale folia)
3 ounces dandelion root (Taraxacum officinale radix)
2 ounces sage (Salvia officinalis)

Take 1 teaspoon in 1 cup of water or herb tea after meals three times a day. The last dose should be taken after dinner or three hours before bedtime to prevent any interference with sleep.

On its own, ginseng can be taken in a variety of ways depending on the quality of the products available and personal preference. For example:

- Dried root: 500 to 2,000 mg daily (can be purchased in 250 mg capsules)
- Tea/infusion: Pour 1 cup boiling water over 1 teaspoon finely chopped ginseng root. Steep for five to ten minutes. Prepare and drink one to three times daily for three to four weeks.
- Tincture (1 : 5): 1 to 2 teaspoons
- Liquid extract (1 : 1): ¼ to ½ teaspoon

SIBERIAN GINSENG

Although part of the same plant family as *Panax ginseng,* Siberian ginseng (*Eleutherococcus senticosus*) is an entirely different plant and does not contain ginsenosides, the active ingredients found in both Asian and American ginseng. *Eleutherococcus,* unlike *Panax,* is not a stimulant or sexual enhancer. But like *Panax,* it is better taken regularly over a period of weeks or months. It may be useful for people who are run-down, weak, lacking in energy and resistance, or suffering from chronic illness. It is especially useful for women whose menopausal symptoms are related to stress. Siberian ginseng can improve sleep, mental performance, stamina, blood-sugar stabilization, and general immune response.

I often recommend Siberian ginseng because it is safe for women who cannot take true ginseng because of high blood pressure, mental illness, or sensitivity to stimulants or certain medications. As always, check with an experienced herbalist or your health-care provider before self-medicating. Siberian ginseng can be taken in a combination formula as above (in place of *Panax ginseng*), or it may be taken on its own.

The Siberian ginseng dose I recommend is 2 to 4 grams of root simmered into a cup of tea, prepared according to the standard directions and taken one to three times a day. The tea can be taken on and off for an indefinite period of time, as needed. The equivalent tincture dose is 1 teaspoon in 1 cup of water, one to four times a day.

SAINT-JOHN'S-WORT

Saint-John's-wort (*Hypericum perforatum*) has been used by herbalists for many years as a treatment for digestive ailments and as a sedative, painkiller, and analgesic. Long before the term *depression* was coined, folk remedies that included Saint-John's-wort were prescribed for common symptoms of depression, including insomnia, anxiety, and nervous unrest.

The herb combines anti-inflammatory, antiviral, and wound-healing properties with a restorative effect on the nerves. Saint-John's-wort also may reduce dependence on painkillers or antidepressants. However, menopausal women on antidepressants should consult with an herbalist and their prescribing physician if they wish to include this herb in addition to or in place of medication.

There has been a lot of attention paid in the media to the dangers of Saint-John's-wort in terms of its interaction with other medications. Of course, it is always important to consult with your doctor or other practitioner about what drugs you are taking and any possible interactions with herbal remedies.

The standard dose is 900 mg per day (300 mg three times a day) or a 5 ml tincture taken three times a day.

KAVA KAVA

Kava kava (*Piper methysticum*), or simply kava for short, is a South Pacific root that is used as a natural sedative and sleep enhancer. Kava may promote a feeling of relaxation, peace, and contentment. As a sleep aid it promotes deep and restful sleep. It is also prescribed for short-term use to reduce anxiety and for hot flashes and mood changes triggered by menopause.

Though it has received negative attention in the press, I have had a lot of success treating menopausal symptoms with kava. The American Botanical Council recommends that kava not be used by anyone who has liver problems, is taking medications with known adverse effects on the liver, or is a regular consumer of alcohol. Kava is not generally recommended for pregnant women or young teens below the age of puberty.

The dose is traditionally in the form of a brewed tea (decoction) of 2 to 3 grams. It can also be taken in capsule form. Be sure the supplement is standardized to contain 30 percent kavalactones. Kava should not be taken for more than four weeks without professional supervision.

CHAMOMILE AND PASSIONFLOWER

Two other herbs used for stress reduction are chamomile (*Matricaria chamomilla*) and passionflower (*Passiflora incarnata*).

Chamomile is a bitter digestive aid and relaxes frazzled nerves. A therapeutic dose of chamomile tea is 1 ounce steeped for fifteen minutes, covered, and taken 1 cup before meals two to four times a day. An equivalent in tincture is 5 ml (1 teaspoon) diluted in water or tea before meals two to four times a day.

Passionflower is often prescribed to treat restlessness, anxiety, and insomnia. It is also used for emotional swings that sometimes occur with physical pain. The herb appears to work, at least in part, by mildly depressing the central nervous system and preventing muscle spasms.

The dosage range for tincture, which is the most effective form, is ½ to 1 teaspoon daily, or ½ to 1½ ounces tincture per week.

Herbs for Hot Flashes and Night Sweats

Hot flashes may respond well to many herbal remedies. As our blood vessels become more sensitive to sharp drops and floods of hormones during menopause, certain herbs can help stabilize blood pressure and reduce hot flashes and night sweats. However, because a person's response to an herb is highly individual, you may have to try several different herbs or herbal formulas before you find one that works for you. The following are a few of the most effective herbs that I use to treat these menopausal symptoms.

BLACK COHOSH

A native American root, black cohosh (*Cimicifuga racemosa*) seems to work by supporting and maintaining the levels of certain female hormones, which may lessen the severity of hot flashes. (Black cohosh should not be taken if a woman is experiencing heavy bleeding.)

The whole root extract of black cohosh has a complex chemistry; it contains isoflavones (phytoestrogens), plant acids, resins, calcium, magnesium, manganese, potassium, and zinc. Taken as a tea or tincture, black cohosh has milder but broader effects than extracts. Vaginal atrophy may be prevented or improved by taking black cohosh. The isoferulic and salicylic acids in black cohosh have a mild, temporary sedative effect on nerves. And clinical studies show the whole root extract acts as a significant antidepressant.[3]

In the 1980s, three controlled trials compared synthetic and conjugated estrogens to both a standardized preparation of black cohosh and a placebo, and all three found the herbal product was often as effective as HRT.[4] A recent trial showed that plant estrogens such as those in black cohosh did not worsen endometrial cancers[5] and in some cases may protect against them.[6] Published trials to date on black cohosh have used varying doses of Remifemin, the standardized extract. The whole herb, black cohosh, has not been studied.

More recently, there has been a media scare regarding cancer metastatis and liver toxicity with the use of black cohosh. The Center for Science in the Public Interest, a private corporation, found evidence that mice with breast cancer who were given black cohosh had spreading of the cancer to the lungs. If you have a history of breast cancer or liver problems, it would be prudent to discuss your use of black cohosh with your health-care providers before starting a regimen.

The tincture dose is ½ to 1 teaspoon (2 to 4 ml) of a 1 : 2 or 1 : 3 extract in water two to three times a day. Commonly, tinctures in retail outlets are 1 : 5, in which case I recommend a higher dose of 7 to 7.5 ml per day. The standardized extract dose is two Remifemin tablets twice a day (20 mg including 1 mg deoxyactein per tablet, or liquid equivalent). Tea or capsule dose is ½ to 1 gram dried root three times a day. It often takes two to six weeks of treatment to decrease symptoms such as night sweats to a manageable level. Herbalists usually prescribe black cohosh in combination with other herbs over the course of many months before tapering off gradually.

The sample formula below combines three tinctures available in many stores and Internet herb shops or by mail order:

SAMPLE TINCTURE FOR HOT FLASHES

2 ounces black cohosh (Cimicifuga racemosa)
1 ounce dandelion leaf (Taraxacum officinale folia)
1 ounce black haw root (Viburnum prunifolium)

Pour the tinctures into a 4-ounce dark glass bottle with a cap and label it immediately with the date, contents, and the following directions: *Take ½ teaspoon two to three times a day, diluted in 3 ounces water.*

It is best to take this formula after meals, but it can be diluted with more water and taken on an empty stomach. Each dose provides 2.5 ml black cohosh tincture; the maximum daily dose is 7.5 ml. Excess black cohosh (more than 20 ml tincture in twenty-four hours) can cause a frontal headache. Sensitive women may start with half the dose: ¼ teaspoon two to three times a day, gradually increasing over two weeks as needed.

MOTHERWORT AND LINDEN FLOWER

Motherwort (*Leonurus cardiaca*) is used in Europe for treating heart palpitations, especially when they are experienced together with hot flashes. It is thought to help liver and cardiac function, and it is a mild nervous system relaxant. Motherwort can relieve hot flashes; improve digestion, including increased absorption of nutrients, vitamins, and herbs; and reduce hormonal or anxiety-triggered heart palpitations.

Concentrated liquid preparations can be taken by the dropperful (approximately 1 ml) every ten minutes, though two doses is usually sufficient. The tea or tincture dose is equivalent to 2 grams taken one to three times a day as needed.

Linden blossom (*Tilia platyphylla* or *T. europea*) mildly reduces elevated blood pressure without any evidence of interacting with blood pressure medications and can calm an upset stomach. Far less bitter than motherwort, linden flower, sometimes called lime flower (no relation to the fruit), has a mildly sweet taste and silky quality that calm a nervous stomach. In the case of nervous upset that affects the stomach and triggers hot flashes, the dose of linden flower in either tea or tincture is equivalent to 2 to 4 grams taken two to four times a day.

Herbs for Insomnia

Interrupted or disturbed sleep, difficulty falling asleep, and problems falling back to sleep during the night are common symptoms of both menopause and aging. The following herbs are the ones I recommend to my patients for a range of sleep issues.

VALERIAN

As a sleep aid, Valerian root (*Valeriana officinalis*) is often combined with one of the following relaxing herbs: the bitter sedative hops (*Humulus lupulus*), skullcap (*Scutellaria galericulata*), passionflower (*Passiflora incarnata*), or the analgesic Jamaican dogwood (*Piscidia erythrina*).

Valerian has been shown to improve the quality of sleep, confirmed to some degree by electroencephalograms (a technology that traces brain waves). Valerian acts by binding with GABA (gamma-aminobutyric acid, a neurotransmitter responsible for relaxation and sleep) receptors. Valerian shortens the time it takes to fall asleep, especially in the elderly and in habitual poor sleepers. It does not cause morning drowsiness. Below is a formula that contains valerian and passionflower, both of which are safe and effective herbs for promoting sleep. Research shows that valerian or combinations containing this herb are most effective when they are taken for a minimum of four to five nights in a row.

INSOMNIA FORMULA

2 ounces valerian root (Valeriana officinalis)
2 ounces passionflower (Passiflora incarnata)

Steep 1 teaspoon of each of the herbs in 1 cup cold water for two hours to extract all the relaxing properties of the herbs without heat, then strain. Drink ⅓ cup one hour before bed, and again at bedtime, or as needed every twenty minutes. Of course, a regular brew of valerian root tea also can help with sleep, but it smells much worse. One alternative is to buy 1-ounce bottles of each herb in tincture form; combine them, then take 1 to 3 teaspoons at bedtime, up to 6 teaspoons each night (6 teaspoons = 1 fluid ounce). Another alternative is to take 500 mg of a soft gel capsule at night.

Herbs for Osteoporosis

The following herbal remedies are not a treatment or proven prevention for osteoporosis on their own, but combined with a healthy diet and regular exercise they can help to ameliorate the onset or lessen the severity of menopausal osteoporosis for some women. Many herbalists consider the following nutritive herbs to be most effective when taken as a tea instead of a tincture because the whole herbs are more beneficial and the water in herb tea assists in absorption.

HERBAL TEA

1½ ounces nettle (Urtica dioica)
1 ounce oatstraw herb (Avena sativa)
1 ounce raspberry leaf (Rubus idaeus)
½ ounce red clover flower (Trifolium pratense)
2 ounces lemon balm herb (Melissa officinalis)

Other herbs to add or substitute, according to your tastes:

Rose hips (*Rosa canina*)	1 ounce	flavor, some bioflavonoids
Alfalfa herb (*Medicago sativa*)	½ ounce	phytoestrogens and minerals
Horsetail herb (*Equisetum arvense*)	½ ounce	may improve mineralization

Mix the chosen herbs together. Pour 1 pint (2 cups) boiling water over 1 ounce of the herb combination (approximately ⅓ cup), and let steep in a covered teapot or container for fifteen minutes. Strain through a tea strainer; drink 2 cups a day, hot or cold. These herbs can also be taken in liquid, tablet, or capsule form.

Herbs for Other Common Menopausal Symptoms

Herbal remedies also can help alleviate other symptoms of menopause such as vaginal atrophy and irregular bleeding that are frequently reported. Interestingly, many of the women I treat find these symptoms even more distressing than hot flashes or the fear of osteoporosis.

VITEX

Vitex (*Vitex agnus-castus*), also called chasteberry or chaste tree, has been central to women's hormonal health in the Western world for three thousand years. Vitex is now known to impact sex steroid levels, although how it does this is only partly understood. Medieval European monks used vitex to lower their libido, hence the name *chaste*berry. Vitex seeds or berries are pungent with low to no toxicity. They contain glycosides, flavonoids, and essential oils.

Traditionally, chasteberry is not used on its own to treat menopausal symptoms. It works best when combined with herbs that assist the body's hepatic and endocrine balance of hormones, such as dandelion, and that relieve muscular tension, such as black haw. Although vitex is commonly described as a progesterone-promoting remedy, some herbalists consider it a healer of the ovarian clock: it regulates the timing of erratic menstrual cycles and may decrease excess estrogen associated with uterine fibroids, fibrocystic breast lumps, and symptoms of PMS.

Clinical trials have shown that the herb is effective in treating early menopause, especially with irregular cycles, with or without PMS. Herbalists also use it when women in perimenopause have PMS, heavy bleeding, or irregular cycles.

Low doses are used in Germany: 40 mg of herb extracted as an infusion or tincture. Elsewhere, the dose is one 500-mg tablet per day, or a tincture ranging from 2 ml of 1:2 tincture to 5 ml of 1:5 (common strength in retail). It is common throughout the monthly cycle to take one daily dose upon rising. In large trials, side effects, mainly nausea, have been minimal (about 1 percent of more than 1,500 women) and temporary.

The following formula delivers optimum amounts of safe, effective hormone-balancing herbs for women who are still menstruating. It is especially effective if your cycles are getting shorter and closer together.

HERBAL FORMULA (EXTRACTS)

2 ounces chasteberry (Vitex agnus-castus)
2 ounces black haw (Viburnum prunifolium)
3 ounces dandelion root (Taraxacum officinale radix)

Combine these extracts and take 1 teaspoon three times a day, plus one dropperful (up to ¼ teaspoon) for symptom relief every ten minutes or as needed. Tea for this formula is also effective. Combine in the same proportions as above, simmer for twenty minutes, strain, and drink ½ to 1 cup twice a day (the taste is slightly bitter). Tea or extracts of these herbs can be used for one to three months.

In traditional herbal medicine, formulas for reproductive health are always rounded out with herbs to nourish the whole woman. In this balanced formula, dandelion supports liver and kidney function. Dandelion leaf and root add nutritive value, with small amounts of easily assimilated vitamins (beta-carotene, vitamin D, and vitamin B-complex) and minerals including iron, magnesium, and zinc. The leaf reduces water retention and bloating. Dandelion's bitter compounds improve the liver's and gall bladder's natural roles in metabolizing fats. While this adds to the formula's postmenopausal protection against heart disease, dandelion leaf and root together improve elimination without any harsh laxative effects. This protects women against constipation and long-term consequences of bowel toxicity, even while dandelion's gentle stimulation of liver function aids each woman's balance of hormones, energy level, and immunity.

BLACK HAW

Black haw (*Viburnum prunifolium*) is an example of an herb that works better as tea than as tincture or tablet, but in all forms it can reduce painful spasms of the uterus and pelvic region. Botanically this herb is related to crampbark (*Viburnum opulus*), which relaxes smooth muscle throughout the body and eases breathing (bronchodilation) and circulation. Increased circulation improves cerebral blood flow (bringing oxygen to the brain), which may help memory. The two herbs are sometimes used interchangeably, although black haw is better for easing cramps.

The relaxing effect of black haw is partly due to the flavonoid amentoflavone, although it also has glycosides, triterpenes, plant acids, coumarins, and other compounds. The pleasant-tasting bark tea or extract may help decrease slightly elevated blood pressure, protecting women against some of the cardiovascular complications linked to postmenopause.[7]

The recommended dose is 2 to 5 grams in capsules, or 1 to 2 teaspoons tincture. If taking as tea, follow the standard preparation (infusion, or steeped fifteen to twenty minutes). Whichever form you choose, take three times a day.

WILD YAM

Wild yam (*Dioscorea villosa*) extract is the base for many natural creams used to treat some menopausal symptoms—particularly creams designed to improve vaginal lubrication. This is more than temporary lubrication;

true herbal creams are used to improve the tone and tissue integrity of the vaginal lining. Sex and/or five minutes a day of Kegel exercises are also naturally stimulating to vaginal lubrication. (An explanation of Kegels can be found in chapter 8.)

Diosgenin, which is a phytoestrogen compound from wild yam that is converted into natural progesterone in a laboratory, was used in early commercial production of the birth control pill and other sex hormones. Wild yam is still used as a precursor in the manufacture of "natural progesterones." Natural progesterone products including Pro-Gest may indeed help reduce hot flashes or improve vaginal health. While the chemical transformation of dioscin (also extracted from wild yam) or diosgenin to estrogen and other steroidal compounds can be accomplished in the laboratory, this conversion does not occur in the human body. Not enough is known about this process to rely on wild yam extracts to protect the uterine linings of women taking estrogen (for a discussion of natural hormones and wild yam, see chapter 5).

DONG QUAI

Dong quai (*Angelica sinensis*) is a member of the fennel and carrot family. The root of the plant is the part used most often for medicinal purposes. The root contains phytosterols, essential oils, coumarins, and other substances that can inhibit blood clotting and improve circulation. Dong quai is known both in China and the West for its ability to support and maintain the natural balance of female hormones. Its traditional uses include treating painful periods, constipation, and other conditions associated with pelvic congestion.

Dong quai is promoted in the U.S. market as a general treatment for women's health. However, recent debate has centered on whether it has estrogenlike effects. Chinese studies as early as 1957 and as recent as 1987 show that it does not. In experimental isolation, it may not be effective as a hot-flash remedy. But in herbal practice, dong quai is given together with other herbs to stimulate sluggish blood flow experienced by some perimenopausal women. In combination with other herbs it may also re-duce hot flashes and night sweats for women in early menopause who still have difficult periods.

Dong quai is rarely prescribed on its own. I encourage you to seek a practitioner of traditional Chinese medicine or herbal medicine who can prescribe a formula that suits your individual symptoms. Because it thins the blood, dong quai should be avoided by women on warfarin (Cou-madin).[8] It is also contraindicated in acute illness, and for women with heavy bleeding or frequent hot flashes with bright-red facial flushing.

RED CLOVER

Red clover (*Trifolium pratense*) is traditionally used by herbalists because it is considered a gentle herb that can alter long-term conditions such as skin problems, arthritis, and degenerative diseases. It assists the body's natural healing through detoxification. It is also nutritive. Recently, red clover has gained attention as a source of isoflavones and is being mar-keted for menopausal symptoms. It does contain isoflavones—substances that have estrogenlike effects similar to soy and black cohosh. Isoflavones have been proven in some studies to have a beneficial effect on blood ves-sels, improving their elasticity in menopausal women and thus reducing hot flashes and night sweats.[9] (For a full discussion of isoflavones, see chapter 5.)

However, clinical studies conducted in the United States and Australia on Promensil, an Australian product containing red clover, have yielded different results. The trials, paid for by the manufacturers of Promensil, found that the isoflavone product was not effective at reducing hot flashes in two studies but it was effective in a third study. In the trial, women who had an average of thirty-five hot flashes a week, even as many as eight a day, tried Promensil, or a similar red clover product, or a placebo. Vegetar-ians, women who eat soy foods, and those on certain medications were ex-cluded from the study because these differences can throw off test results.

The women took the products for three months—long enough to

have some effect but probably not long enough to determine safety. The researchers concluded that there was not a large enough difference among Promensil, the other red clover product Rimostil, and the placebo to show that these isoflavone products reduced hot flashes. Yet they did see a reasonable biological basis for the way red clover isoflavones might affect menopausal women.[10]

Traditional herbal medicine does not use the whole herb red clover to treat hot flashes (such large amounts would have to be taken that women would have to eat bales of it). Instead, it is used in a tincture, extract, or tea form. Red clover's main effects include improving lymphatic flow, hence possibly clearing acne, reducing joint pains, and lightening menstrual periods.

Red clover also has long been used to treat breast cancer. One of red clover's phytoestrogen constituents, biochanin-A, inhibits carcinogen activation in cells. The drug tamoxifen, used to treat breast cancer, is structurally related to the phytoestrogens. However, the effect of regular use of red clover products based on isoflavones by women who already have, or have had, estrogen-dependent cancer requires further long-term study.

HRT and Herbal Treatment Combinations

Most of the herbs mentioned in this chapter can be taken safely by women who are on conventional hormone therapies. If you want to try herbs but your doctor cannot answer your questions, find a qualified herbalist, or see a naturopath, nurse-practitioner, certified nurse midwife (CNM), or other care provider who is trained in women's preventive health.

If you've been taking estrogen or estrogen-progesterone therapy and have decided to stop, it is not necessary to wean off slowly (strictly speaking), but some say doing so helps prevent the return of symptoms, especially hot flashes and mood changes. Many women start adding herbal treatments as they're decreasing their dosage of the conventional hormones. It is prudent to consider regular medical monitoring during this time.

Here is my advice for ways to slowly taper off hormone therapy:

1. Take the lowest dose that controls symptoms on Day 1 through Day 25, then your regular dose for the next seven to ten days.
2. For the first month, use herbs recommended by your health-care provider, or try the tincture or the tea formula for black cohosh discussed earlier, without changing your HRT dose.
3. During the second month, reduce the dose of HRT by a quarter.
4. As your body adjusts to the withdrawal of supplemental estrogen, there may be a few symptoms. Adjust your herbal tea accordingly—drink it slightly stronger or more frequently to counteract symptoms. If your symptoms are severe, go back to the full HRT dose plus the herbs, for an extra month or more, until you and your health-care provider feel ready to try again. If, however, all is going well, reduce HRT from the three-quarter dose to half dose in the third month. Continue dietary improvements, herbs, and exercise recommendations as you slowly reduce your HRT dose, a quarter at a time.
5. Skip one day per week of a cyclical drug program. Then every month, drop another quarter dose while using an herbal preparation recommended by your health-care provider.
6. When you are only taking a quarter of your original HRT dose along with the herbs, take the pills only every other day, then every third day.
7. As you feel ready (health signs stay stable as drugs are slowly reduced), skip an extra day each week until you are taking the hormones only once a week.
8. After three to six months, wean off HRT completely and reassess. Even though some initial symptoms or signs (such as bone loss, rebound hot flashes) may temporarily return, they should be minimal.
9. Use herbs if needed up to an additional three to six months.

TIPS FOR TAPERING

- If you are having problems, reevaluate your nutritional choices, stress-reduction techniques, and other lifestyle factors.
- You can drop the dosage at any rate, but try to do it with consistency and rhythm.
- If you're not feeling well at any time, increase your dosage to the last amount that felt comfortable.

Loreen's Story

Loreen is fifty-four and married, with two grown children. She owns her own business and has always enjoyed life. Loreen had been on an HRT Premarin/progesterone regimen for eight years, and her periods were a "major hassle." She slept poorly, waking frequently with hot flashes. Her energy dropped during the day, and she was often depressed.

She decided to adopt a more "natural" HRT therapy. Unfortunately, she dropped the Premarin cold turkey, which is not advisable. When she went off the Premarin, her symptoms—especially the depression—initially improved, but within one month the hot flashes and other symptoms had returned, and they were even more intense. So Loreen went back on Premarin. But this time she decided she needed help and she came to see me.

Loreen's diet was fairly balanced and she did get some cardiovascular exercise, although not enough. She just needed to make a few adjustments. My recommendations:

- Step up exercise program from three to four days a week.
- Eat more beans (in soups, purées, vegetable dips) as a protein substitute for red meat, and replace processed-sugar snacks with small servings of organic nuts and dried fruits.
- Add specific herbal treatments.

In terms of the herbal remedies, I recommended a 4-ounce tincture combining 1 ounce each of passionflower (*Passiflora incarnata*), black cohosh (*Cimicifuga racemosa*), fenugreek (*Trigonella foenum-graecum*), and sage leaf (*Salvia officinalis*). I made sure they were all 1:2 strength extracts. The ratio (1:2) is important because these tinctures are offered only by a professional practitioner and are about two and a half times stronger than retail tinctures. Loreen took 2 milliliters (about ½ teaspoon) in water four times a day, or more as needed.

At first Loreen objected to the bitter taste of the herbs, but after the first three days she began to associate the taste with feeling better. Three weeks later, on her second visit, Loreen reported she had fewer night sweats and hot flashes. She felt mentally and emotionally balanced, even with heavy pressures at work. We repeated the above formula and scheduled an appointment in four weeks.

After a total of seven weeks on the formula, Loreen still complained of symptoms, but they were less severe. She was sleeping better and she felt good about what she was doing. For her next formula, I gave her *Cimicifuga* 1:2 (3 ounces), *Salvia* 1:2 (3 ounces), and *Leonotis leonurus* (wild dagga) 1:2 (4 ounces). She could take 2.5 to 5 ml as needed, three to six times per day. Her annual physical was coming; we agreed she would have a complete blood count (CBC), a bone scan, and the usual tests for her age group, and inform her physician of her herb use. All test results reflected the health "of a thirty-year-old." Loreen was proud she'd accomplished something that her doctor thought was "too hazardous" the previous year.

Loreen checked in with me by phone after that. We adjusted her formula after the first three months, reducing the formula by one dose per day every week over a final two months, and then dropped the herbs altogether without incident. In five months, Loreen felt better, had no symptoms, and was no longer reliant on standard HRT or herbs.

Conclusion

Each menopausal woman is healed when she chooses her own way, whether it be botanical support or the use of hormones to improve her quality of life. Taking hormones for menopause, whether from pregnant mares' urine (Premarin), pharmaceutically altered wild yam roots ("natural" progesterone), or even the popular DHEA, are all options for women today. Yet another option is to choose foods and whole, unadulterated herbs with a traditional affinity for easing a natural rite of change. To be empowered means each woman will decide for herself what serves her highest good. All treatments, botanical or medical, have value if they bring a woman well-being to fulfill her potential.

4 Managing Menopause with Traditional Chinese Medicine

Isaac Cohen, OMD, L.Ac.

Isaac Cohen, a practitioner for seventeen years, is one of the leading authorities in the field of women's health and traditional Chinese medicine. A pioneer in work designed to provide scientific translation of traditional Chinese medical concepts and therapies, Dr. Cohen lectures internationally on the integration of traditional Chinese medicine (TCM) to treat women's diseases. He was one of the founders of the complementary and alternative medicine program at the Carol Franc Buck Breast Care Center at the University of California, San Francisco, and has an ongoing relationship with the Chinese Society for the Integration of TCM and Western Medicine for the Prevention and Treatment of Cancer, in Beijing. Dr. Cohen has a doctorate in Oriental medicine from the Postgraduate Institute of Oriental Medicine in Hong Kong and has trained with the most renowned cancer specialists in China. He has spearheaded clinical and laboratory research at the University of California, San Francisco, to assess the efficacy of herbal therapies for menopause and cancer and to discover mechanistic explanations for the clinical application of natural products. He is currently the chief executive officer of Bionovo, Inc., in Emeryville, California, a drug discovery and development company that focuses on women's health.

When I first started practicing medicine I had vast theoretical knowledge of diseases and their symptoms. However, I was very young and very healthy, and my own experience of illness and suffering was drawn only from having had a cold or mild fever. As a young, conscientious practitioner I tried very hard to relate to symptoms and imagine how it might actually feel to experience them myself. The majority of women who came to see me with menopausal symptoms were women who were taking hormone replacement therapy and were thinking of getting off of it, or those who were just beginning to have unbearable symptoms but feared taking hormones.

I remember that at first I had some trouble empathizing with many of my patients' suffering. The lack of sleep I remembered from when I was in the military. But the rest—the hot flashes, the night sweats, the memory loss—I just didn't know what these women were feeling. Then one day something happened that changed the way I related to and treated my patients—I finally got what a hot flash is.

I was sitting in my office with one of my female patients who had been having severe menopausal symptoms—especially hot flashes. We were talking about her condition; she was explaining, and I was listening and asking questions. Then, I noticed she was getting a bit edgy and irritable. Beads of sweat were forming on her upper lip. Her neck and chest were becoming red, and she looked like she was being baked. As a young, naïve physician I asked the obvious: "Are you having a hot flash right now?" Her answer was something like "Duh."

The Traditional Chinese Medicine Approach to Menopause

Chinese medical tradition views menopause as an important but transitional time in a woman's life cycle—a time of great possibility, but also a time when her energy and normal body/mind functions are in a state of flux, leaving her vulnerable to various symptoms such as hot flashes, sleep disturbances, and depression.

According to traditional Chinese medicine, reproductive function is governed by the kidneys. Sufficient energy in a woman's kidneys is necessary for fertility, libido, regeneration of the entire body, and tissue elasticity and strength. At puberty, a woman's kidney energy increases, sending excess blood to the uterus. During her reproductive years, a woman's kidneys supply enough blood for fertility, but as she ages, the blood flow from her kidneys diminishes, leading to menopause. Menopausal problems occur when kidney energy is depleting and cannot sustain all of the rest of the body's vital functions.

During this time, the body's vital life energy, or qi (in particular, the kidney energy) is low and going through reorganization and resource management for safe aging. It is a positive change that takes time and some pain to accomplish. The end result is that although the reproductive toll is far greater on a woman's body than on a man's, women generally end up living longer because of this resource management.

Because of menstruation and childbearing, women lose a large amount of blood during their lives. From a Chinese medicine point of view, the blood is never completely replenished—not in volume and not in quality. In China, menstrual blood loss is considered to be a major contributing factor in chronic diseases and aging. Since aging is viewed as physical and functional deterioration of the body, chronic loss of blood is thought to contribute to the deterioration process. Some of the functional difficulties that occur during menopause such as sleep disturbance, mood changes, dry skin, and vaginal dryness are thought to be directly related to the decline in blood nourishing these tissues. And the time right before menopause is when women experience these changes most dramatically.

Women often complain of exhaustion and confusion during perimenopause and early menopause. In Chinese medicine this is attributed to a depletion of the spirit, or "shen," which governs mental processes—the mind's ability to think, form ideas, and maintain awareness. More specifically, shen is a measurement of vitality, and the quality of that vitality is best seen in a person's eyes. The loss of shen that occurs around the years leading up to menopause can result in memory loss, inability to think straight, mood swings, and insomnia. Some of this cognitive change is reversed when the menopausal process is complete, and some of it is more permanent. For example, at the onset of menopause many women experience acute problems with concentration that seem to get better after a while. However, short-term memory loss that comes with menopause seems to stay with women. In Chinese medicine we may use herbs or acupuncture to calm the heart and nurture the spirit in order to address or prevent these symptoms.

Chinese medicine attributes particular changes that women experience during menopause to a function of a particular organ. For example, if a woman's body is not transforming food into the necessary nutrients, Chinese medical practitioners will say that the spleen is not functioning properly (this is very different from what the spleen's function is in Western medicine). In my experience, a woman whose spleen is not functioning properly may have weaker hot flashes with more sweating and clamminess.

Another important function of the kidneys in Chinese medicine is the control of water, the substrate for life's activities and the whole of moisture in the body. The kidneys regulate the fluid balance in the channels, blood vessels, and tissues. The function of water regulation in Chinese medicine is accomplished by kidney fire (the kidneys' function in the maintenance of the body's heat). The kidneys are very closely associated with the body's thermal regulation. Too much, not enough, or improper regulation results in sensations of cold or shivers, heat or feverishness, and, during menopause, hot flashes and night sweats.

In Chinese medicine, the variations in the menstrual cycle during perimenopause are a direct result of the degree and type of kidney debilitation. The depletion of kidney reserves happens gradually, in synch with perimenopause and then menopause itself.

Traditional Chinese Medicine Versus Western Medicine

Western society has only recently begun to recognize old age as a valuable time in our lives. This is in part because our life expectancy has increased: Many of us will now live more than a third of our lives in the senior years. Also, it is a recent revelation for Westerners that how we treat our bodies today has an effect on how we might feel and how healthy we are tomorrow (and the day after). This is not a new concept in Chinese medicine, however. This focus on health maintenance and disease prevention throughout life is the foundation of Chinese medicine.

There are many differences in approach between Chinese and Western medicine. One of the major differences is that Chinese medicine treats disease by considering the body as a single functioning unit and symptoms as a reflection of the health of the body as a whole. Whereas Western medicine tends to focus primarily on the specific complaint (for example, hot flashes) and then on treating the suspected "cause" (in this case, the decline in reproductive hormones), it often does so to the exclusion of overall health.

For example, one of the goals of Chinese medicine in treating hot flashes is to prevent any serious complications such as cancer recurrence, heart disease, and osteoporosis that might result from the treatment itself. The safety and effectiveness of treating menopause with estrogen and progesterone, the two most common reproductive hormones prescribed by Western doctors, has recently been called into question. Today, HRT is contraindicated for many women, including those with certain pre-existing conditions such as breast cancer, stroke, recent heart attack, tendency for blood clotting, diabetes, gallbladder disease, high blood pressure, and uterine fibroids, among others.[1-3] Still, for these women, Western medicine has little more to offer them by way of treatment options. There are many alternatives available that are effective for treating the symptoms of menopause. Unfortunately, a woman is unlikely to hear about them from her doctor.

As a Chinese medicine specialist and licensed acupuncturist, I have been treating women for menopausal symptoms for decades. During these years, I have treated a significant number of women with a history of breast cancer. A very high percentage of the women with breast cancer experience severe menopausal symptoms. This is because a woman who is premenopausal at the time of her breast cancer diagnosis is very likely to go into early menopause if she is treated with chemotherapy and/or tamoxifen (a hormone treatment for breast cancer). In these cases, my first priority is to find a way to treat the symptoms without increasing the chance of recurrence.

In Chinese medicine, there is no one treatment for a condition such as menopause. The method of treatment changes for each woman during the course of her therapy, depending on her symptoms—whether they improve or worsen. Seasonal changes may also affect the course of treatment. For instance, most women who suffer from hot flashes due to menopause find they worsen during the summer months. Chinese practitioners understand this and will make accommodations by altering treatment at the end of the spring. Treatment also needs to respond to the changing seasons of life: As a woman ages, treatment may have to be modified on a regular basis. This constant modification means there is much less risk of long-term complications from the treatment itself since most of the time the increased risk from medications is a result of overdosing or prolonged exposure.

In Chinese medicine, instead of automatically writing one prescription for menopausal symptoms, we tailor a specific therapy to both alleviate the symptoms and treat any pre-existing conditions. In other words, we make the treatment fit the individual woman rather than the other way around. For instance, one woman may have hot flashes accompanied by weak vision, dizziness, night sweats, and restless sleep. Another patient may have low back pain, memory problems, and vaginal dryness along with the hot flashes. One of these women may notice that she feels sad and cries easily, whereas the other may get angry and frustrated. Both of these patients will be treated with different acupuncture points, different nutritional advice, and different herbs.

In this chapter I will describe the causes of menopause as described in Chinese medicine and the many treatments available to women, such as acupuncture and herbal remedies. The information and treatment suggestions are derived from the ancient literature, current scientific investigations, and my experience as a clinician.

This chapter is not meant as a substitute for seeing a traditional Chinese medicine practitioner. It is meant to be used as a general guide to the wealth of resources Chinese medicine has to offer. Specific treatments will vary depending on a range of individual factors. Because no two people's symptoms are exactly the same, no two treatment plans will be exactly alike. For this reason and others, it is important not to self-medicate when it comes to herbal remedies. My ultimate goal in this chapter is to provide you with the information and instill in you the confidence that, with the help of a practitioner, you can safely and effectively manage your menopausal symptoms.

Hot Flashes

A hot flash is a sudden surge of heat felt on the face, neck, shoulders, and chest, lasting several minutes or more. It may be preceded or accompanied by a rapid heartbeat and sweating, nausea, dizziness, anxiety, headache, weakness, or a feeling of suffocation. Some women experience an uneasy feeling just before the hot flash that lets them know it is coming; for others it comes without a warning. (Hot flashes that occur at night are called night sweats.) About 75 percent of women in early menopause experience significant hot flashes. Among all the symptoms of perimenopause and menopause, hot flashes are by far the most uncomfortable and inconvenient for the women who experience them.

Human bodies maintain their temperature in a very narrow range of only about three degrees; between 96 and 99 degrees Fahrenheit is considered normal body temperature. Above 99 degrees is a fever. Below 96 degrees is hypothermic. Temperature is maintained within this narrow range so that your body can function optimally. Your body spends a lot of energy to maintain proper temperature. Some of the mechanisms the body employs to maintain its basal temperature are sweating, changing heartbeat and respiration rates, changing fluid pressure and distribution in the tissues, and activating hormonal pathways. The central nervous system and the brain control this coordinated effort.

It is not known exactly what causes hot flashes. However, hot flashes are considered a thermal irregularity. It would seem that the brain's thermostat is malfunctioning, perhaps due to the natural decline in estrogen during menopause. This decline affects the temperature control center of the brain. The body reacts to cool down the body and release heat by increasing blood flow to the surface of the skin. This increased blood flow to the surface of the skin visibly appears as a flush. A sensation of heat is experienced, along with perspiration, and often a speeding of the heart, followed by a drop in body temperature. A hot flash is often followed by a chill due to the drop in body temperature. Warmer temperatures, stress, spicy foods, as well as caffeine and alcohol all can trigger hot flashes. Hot flashes can be especially bad during the summer months.

The number, duration, time of day, and intensity of hot flashes vary among women. Most women experience the bulk of their hot flashes in the evening near the time they go to sleep and again at dawn. Some women sweat and some don't. Some women have flashes lasting just a few seconds and others experience a thirty-minute ordeal. For some women, it is their head that boils; others feel a prickling in their chest. A sudden severe episode can be frightening; you might even confuse the flash with a heart attack. Most women experience hot flashes for an average period of two to five years, although some women don't experience them at all. Others have hot flashes from perimenopause until their eighties.

Research shows that traditional Chinese medicine including acupuncture and herbs can decrease and often eliminate hot flashes as well as offer significant relief to other menopausal symptoms. Because hot flashes are related to both reproductive changes and aging, and because they tend to stop naturally as time passes, Chinese medicine focuses on the strength of the kidneys or kidney qi in regard to treatment.

TREATING HOT FLASHES WITH ACUPUNCTURE

The basic foundation of acupuncture and Chinese medicine, in general, is that there is a life energy flowing through the body called qi. This energy flows through the body on channels known as meridians that connect all of our major organs (see figure 2). According to Chinese medical theory, illness arises when the cyclical flow of qi in the meridians becomes unbalanced or blocked.

Therefore, the goal of acupuncture is to clear this blocked energy. During the acupuncture treatment, tiny needles are placed along the meridians in your legs, arms, shoulders, or elsewhere. The needles are so thin that most people hardly feel them as they penetrate the skin. Acupuncture points to treat the emotional and physical effects of menopause are located all over the body. The mechanism by which acupuncture reduces hot flashes is unclear. It is widely known that acupuncture can regulate various neurochemicals in the brain, as well as hormonal levels in the blood, which most likely have an effect on thermoregulation.

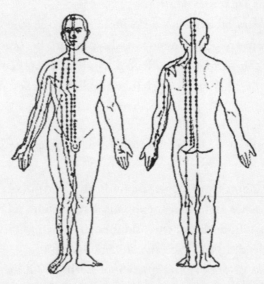

Figure 2: Traditional Chinese Medicine Acupuncture Meridians

The length, number, and frequency of treatments vary. Typical treatments last from five to thirty minutes and may be done one or two times a week. Some symptoms are relieved after the first treatment, while more severe or chronic ailments often require multiple treatments. There are many studies that prove the effectiveness of acupuncture in the treatment of menopausal symptoms. With weekly treatment, the average effect of acupuncture on hot flashes is about 60 percent symptom relief. However, acupuncture treatment has to be ongoing in order to have this dramatic effect.

I have many patients tell me that each acupuncture treatment reduces their symptoms but that symptoms gradually return. How long it takes for the symptoms to return varies depending on the woman. Therefore, I try to determine with each woman on an individual basis how long it usually takes for her symptoms to become bothersome again, and we schedule follow-up treatments accordingly. In the beginning, I recommend having acupuncture treatments more frequently—perhaps a treatment a week for four to eight weeks. After that, the treatments begin to have a cumulative effect, and I may recommend that a patient come to see me once every other week for a few months and then once a month until symptoms are under control.

Over the years of working with women, I've learned to anticipate when and why my patients' menopausal symptoms become worse. Often the severity of the symptoms is affected by physical and emotional issues such as family or work stress or changes in diet and exercise routines.

TREATING HOT FLASHES WITH CHINESE HERBS

In traditional Chinese medicine, many herbal formulas reportedly can alleviate hot flashes and other menopausal symptoms such as insomnia, mood changes, fatigue, headache, and menstrual irregularities including intermittent bleeding and excessive uterine bleeding.

The method of prescribing medicinal herbs in Chinese medicine is very complex. It is rare that a single herb is prescribed by itself; an herbal formula is designed to address the complexity of an individual's condition. Rarely do we use the precise formula studied in a clinical trial or the exact formulation written in our medical textbooks. In practice, formulas are prescribed to each woman on the basis of her individual symptoms and history, and are chosen by the practitioners on the basis of their knowledge of herbs, clinical experience, and intuition.

The physician selects a traditionally prescribed formula that most resembles the woman's condition and then modifies it to suit her symptoms exactly. A traditional formula has any number of ingredients— anywhere from four to eighteen different herbs. It typically contains one to three herbs that treat the specific symptom, one to three herbs that enhance that effect or direct it to specific tissues, and additional herbs that mitigate known side effects or toxicities of the main herbs.

In traditional Chinese medicine, herbal formulas for treating hot flashes—such as Two-Immortal Decoction, Six-Ingredient Pill with Rehmannia, and Geng Nian Fang formula, discussed in the formula guide section of this chapter—are used to treat the whole person, not just to relieve a specific symptom.

There are four principles of diagnosis in Chinese medicine: questioning, observing, listening, and feeling. I also draw on a three-thousand-year-old tradition. My diagnosis might depend upon what a woman says to me, how she acts (for example, if she is agitated or fatigued), how she feels when I palpate her pulse or her abdomen, or even what her tongue looks like.

When I prescribe formulas to treat menopausal symptoms, I do so based on signs and symptoms that I observe. For example, if a woman is complaining of hot flashes, I would recommend a formula based on the specific hot flash experience, such as whether the flashes last for a long time or are brief, come with or without sweats, are accompanied by a mood change, or are followed by chills. I will also check for other health conditions, such as whether the patient has urinary incontinence, is constipated, or has an increased libido.

In the West, there are two Chinese herbs that are promoted to women for almost anything that ails them. These herbs are dong quai (*Angelica sinensis*) and ginseng (*Panax ginseng*). These two herbs are commonly used by women for alleviating menopausal symptoms such as hot flashes and fatigue, although in Chinese medicine they are rarely used to treat menopause.

Some limited research provides conflicting results on the safety and effectiveness of herbal products—such as ginseng, black cohosh, and dong quai—that are marketed for menopausal symptoms. However, herbal products containing or acting like estrogens may provide some of the benefits of estrogen in relieving menopausal symptoms. Currently, the National Institutes of Health's National Center for Complementary and Alternative Medicine (NCCAM) is funding research on several botanicals for reducing menopausal symptoms, including black cohosh, red clover, hops, dong quai, flaxseed, and dietary soy.

FORMULA GUIDE FOR HOT FLASHES

Below are twenty different herbal treatments (or formulas) that are used in Chinese medicine. They are categorized according to the type of hot flashes a woman may experience. I have also included the formal Chinese diagnosis and ways to modify each formula to individualize it.

The formulas are written in the format used by herbal pharmacies: The pinyin Chinese transliteration name is first, and then the pharmacological name (rather than the botanical name) of the herbs. The formulas are meant to be used for two to three months at the most. Once your symptoms are under control, your practitioner may suggest a different formula to address the underlying cause of menopause and to promote a healthy, graceful aging. The dosages are in grams, and each formula is meant for two days of use with 1 cup of the water extract of the formula each day. Most formulas are made as tea unless otherwise indicated. I recommend that you consult a practitioner of Chinese herbal medicine before using any of these formulas.

Following is a list of the most common plant parts and natural products, as well as their abbreviations as they appear in the formulas.

Plant part	Abbreviation
Root	Rx
Rhizome	Rz
Flower	Fl
Fruit	Fr
Seed	Sn
Whole plant	Hb
Bark	Cx
Shell	Os
Twig	Rm
Peel	Per

1. Hot Flashes That Are Worse When You Are Under Stress

OTHER SYMPTOMS: pelvic pain, pain under the diaphragm, dry mouth and throat, fatigue, dry brittle skin, painful swollen breasts

CHINESE DIAGNOSIS: liver constrained with blood deficiency

RECOMMENDED FORMULA: *Rambling Powder Modified—Jia Wei Xiao Yao San*

Yin chai hu	Rx Stellaria dichotoma	15 g
Dong quai	Rx Angelica sinensis	15 g
Bai shao	Rx Paeonia lactiflora	15 g
Bai zhu	Rx Atractylodes macrocephala	15 g
Fu ling	Sclerotium poria cocos (fungus)	15 g
Zhi gan cao	Rx Glycyrrhiza uralensis, honey-fried	8 g
Gou qi zi	Fr Lycii	15 g
Ju hua	Fl Chrysanthemi	15 g
Huai niu xi	Rx Achyranthis	15 g
Bo he	Hb Mentha	6 g

MODIFICATIONS:

Vaginal discharge with vaginal dryness:

Jin yin hua	Fl Lonicera japonica	add 20 g
Ku shen	Rx Sophora flavecentis	add 15 g
Zhi gan cao	Rx Glycyrrhiza uralensis, honey-fried	omit 8 g

Fibrocystic breast with lumps and pain:

Zhi gan cao	Rx Glycyrrhiza uralensis, honey-fried	omit 8 g
Wang bu liu xing	Sn Vaccaria	add 10 g
Ji xue teng	Rx Caulis millettiae seu spatholobi	add 20 g

Heartburn and acid reflux:

Hai piao xiao	Os Sepia seu sepiella	add 12 g
Bie jia	Os Carapax amydae sinensis	add 15 g
Bai zhu	Rx Atractylodes macrocephala	reduce to 8 g

2. Hot Flashes Accompanied by Heavy Sweating and Followed by a Cold Sensation

OTHER SYMPTOMS: nervousness, fatigue, lassitude, depression, irritability, insomnia, palpitations, frequent urination, hypertension

CHINESE DIAGNOSIS: kidney yin and yang deficiency accompanied by flaring up of deficient fire

RECOMMENDED FORMULA: *Two-Immortal Decoction—Er Xian Tang*

Xian mao	Rz Curculiginis orchioidis	6–15 g
Yin yang huo	Hb Epimedi	10–15 g
Ba ji tian	Rx Morinda officinalis	10 g
Huang bai	Cx Phellodendri	5–10 g
Zhi mu	Rx Anemarrhena	5–10 g
Dong quai	Rx Angelica sinensis	10 g

MODIFICATIONS:

For more severe nervousness:

Fu xiao mai	Fr Tritici levis	add 15–20 g
Shi chang pu	Rz Acori graminei	add 8 g

With more severe insomnia:

Yin yang huo	Hb Epimedi	8–15 g
Ban xia	Rz Pinellia ternata	add 8 g
Hu po	Succinum	add 1–2 g
	(resin from pine tree)	

Breast pain and hard nodules and cold sensation in nipples:

Mo yao	Myrrh (resin from spiny deciduous tree)	add 10 g
Gou qi zi	Fr Lycii	add 10–15 g

Pain during intercourse:

Ai ye	Hb Agrimonia	add 10–12 g
Rou cong rong	Hb Cistanches deserticola	add 10 g
She chuang zi	Sn Cnidii monnieri	add 6–10 g

3. Hot Flashes (Mainly Chest and Head) That Are Worse When You Are Tired and Not Eating

OTHER SYMPTOMS: chest pain and hypochondriac pain, chronic stubborn migrainelike headache, depression, restless sleep, irritability, extreme mood swings, suffocating sensation

CHINESE DIAGNOSIS: blood stasis in the chest with impairment of blood flow in the area above the diaphragm

RECOMMENDED FORMULA: *Drive Out Stasis in the Mansion of Blood Decoction—Xue Fu Zhu Yu Tang*

Tao ren	Sn Persica	12 g
Hong hua	Fl Carthami tinctori	10 g
Dong quai	Rx Angelica sinensis	10 g
Chuan xiong	Rx Ligustici wallichii	5 g
Chi shao	Rx Paeonia rubra	6 g

Chuan niu xi	Rx Cyathula officinalis	10 g
Chai hu	Rx Bupleuri	3 g
Jie geng	Rx Platycodi grandiflori	5 g
Zhi ke	Fr Citri seu ponciri	6 g
Sheng di huang	Rx Rehmannia glutinosa	10 g
Gan cao	Rx Glycyrrhiza uralensis	3 g

MODIFICATIONS:
Headache:

| Man jing zi | Fr Viticis | add 10 g |
| Bai ji li | Fr Tribuli terrestris | add 10 g |

Stomach and rib tension:

| Yu jin | Rz Curcuma | add 10 g |
| Wu yao | Rx Lindera strychnifolia | add 10 g |

More chest pain:

| Dan shen | Rx Salvia miltiorrhiza | add 10–15 g |

Hip pain:

| Sang ji sheng | Rm Loranthi seu visci | add 10–20 g |
| Du zhong | Cx Eucommia | add 10 g |

4. Hot Flashes That Are Stronger After Dark and/or Right When You Go to Sleep

OTHER SYMPTOMS: warm palms, dry mouth and lips, no desire to drink, flatulence, depression

CHINESE DIAGNOSIS: deficiency and cold of the ren and chong channels together with blood stasis

RECOMMENDED FORMULA: *Warm the Mensis Decoction—Wen Jing Tang*

Wu zhu yu	Fr Evodia	10 g
Gui zhi	Rm Cinnamomi cassia	6 g
Dong quai	Rx Angelica sinensis	10 g
Chuan xiong	Rx Ligustici wallichii	6 g
Bai shao	Rx Paeonia lactiflora	6 g
E jiao	Gelatinum corii asini (donkey-hide gelatin)	6 g
Mai men dong	Rx Ophiopogonis	10 g
Mu dan pi	Cx Moutan radicis	6 g
Ren shen	Rx Ginseng	6 g
Gan cao	Rx Glycyrrhiza uralensis	6 g
Sheng jiang	Rz Zingiberis officinalis	6 g
Ban xia	Rz Pinellia ternata	6 g

MODIFICATIONS:

Severe gas and bloating:

Wu yao	Rx Lindera strychnifolia	add 10 g
Xiang fu	Rz Cyperi rotundi	add 10 g

Fatigue:

Huang qi	Rx Astragali membranacei	add 10 g

Constipation:

Rou cong rong	Hb Cistanches deserticola	add 10 g

Low libido:

Yin yang huo	Hb Epimedi	add 10–15 g
Bu gu zhi	Fr Psoralea	add 8 g

5. Hot Flashes and Night Sweats That Are Worse At Night

OTHER SYMPTOMS: irritability, overthinking while unable to think straight or concentrate, forgetfulness, insomnia, restless sleep

CHINESE DIAGNOSIS: yin deficiency of the heart and kidney

RECOMMENDED FORMULA: *Emperor of Heaven's Special Pill to Tone the Heart—Tian Wang Bu Xin Dan*

Sheng di huang	Rx Rehmannia glutinosa	120 g
Ren shen	Rx Ginseng	15 g
Tian men dong	Rx Asparagi	30 g
Mai men dong	Rx Ophiopogonis	30 g
Xuan shen	Rx Scrophularia	15 g
Dan shen	Rx Salvia miltiorrhiza	15 g
Fu ling	Sclerotium poria cocos (fungus)	15 g
Yuan zhi	Rx Polygala	15 g
Dong quai	Rx Angelica sinensis	30 g
Wu wei zi	Fr Schizandra	30 g
Bai zi ren	Sn Biota	30 g
Suan zao ren	Sn Zizyphi spinosa	30 g
Jie geng	Rx Platycodi grandiflori	15 g

MODIFICATIONS:

Severe insomnia:

Long yan rou	Fr Arillus longanae	add 10 g
Ye jiao teng	Rx Caulis polygoni multiflori	add 10 g
Ren shen	Rx Ginseng	omit 15 g

Mouth and tongue sores:

Lian zi xin	Fl Plumula nelumbinis	add 15 g

Severe dry mouth and throat:

Shi hu	Hb Dendrobi	add 12 g
Jie geng	Rx Platycodi grandiflori	omit 15 g

Severe mood swings:

Long gu	Os Draconis	add 12 g
Mu li	Concha ostrea (oyster shell)	add 12 g

6. Hot Flashes Mainly in the Chest Accompanied by Severe Irritability and Sense of Exhaustion; Palpitations with Anxiety

OTHER SYMPTOMS: inability to calm down or calmly lie down, insomnia, mouth and tongue sores

CHINESE DIAGNOSIS: yin deficiency fire with fluid damage causing heart and kidney to miscommunicate

RECOMMENDED FORMULA: *Coptis and Donkey-Hide Gelatin Decoction—Huang Lian E Jiao Tang*

Huang lian	Rz Coptidis	12 g
Huang qin	Rx Scutellaria	6 g
E jiao	Gelatinum corii asini (donkey-hide gelatin)	10 g
Bai shao	Rx Paeonia lactiflora	6 g
Ji zi huang	Egg yolks (stir into formula)	2 yolks

MODIFICATIONS:
Severe yin deficiency with fluid damage and a dry throat:

Xuan shen	Rx Scrophularia	add 12 g
Mai men dong	Rx Ophiopogonis	add 12 g
Shi hu	Hb Dendrobi	add 12 g

Heat sensation in palms and soles:

Zhi zi	Fr Gardenia	add 8 g
Dan zhu ye	Hb Lophatheri	add 12 g

7. Hot Flashes That Feel Like They Are Constant, All Day and Night (More Than Fifteen a Day)

OTHER SYMPTOMS: disorientation, frequent attacks of melancholy, crying spells, restless sleep, frequent bouts of yawning, depression, vaginal dryness

CHINESE DIAGNOSIS: restless organ disorder (zang zao); excessive worry, anxiety, or pensiveness that injures the heart yin, which in turn affects liver qi and spleen qi

RECOMMENDED FORMULA: *Licorice, Wheat, and Jujube Decoction— Gan Mai Da Zao Tang*

Gan cao	Rx Glycyrrhiza uralensis	10 g
Fu xiao mai	Sn Tritici levis	10–20 g
Da zao	Fr Jujube	10 pieces

MODIFICATIONS:
Severe night sweats:

Zhi mu	Rx Anemarrhena	add 15 g

Severe fatigue and heat in the chest, irritability:

Bai he	Bulb Lilli	add 12 g
Bai zi ren	Sn Biota	add 12 g

For irritability at night:

Suan zao ren	Sn Zizyphi spinosa	add 12 g

For constipation:

Hei zhi ma	Sn Sesami	add 15 g
He shou wu	Rx Polygoni multiflori	add 12 g

For severe sweating from head, due to food stagnation:

Jiang zhi chao huang lian	Rz Coptidis, ginger-fried	add 8 g
Shan zha	Fr Crataegi	add 10–15 g

For nausea due to food stagnation:

Lian qiao	Fr Forsythia	add 3–8 g
Fu ling	Sclerotium poria cocos (fungus)	add 10–12 g

8. Hot Flashes That Are Caused and/or Accompanied by Fright and by Change of Physical Position

OTHER SYMPTOMS: palpitations, fullness in the chest, feeling of extreme heaviness throughout the body, constipation, stiffness at the waist, urinary difficulty

CHINESE DIAGNOSIS: phlegm in the liver and gallbladder due to damage to fluids and yang qi constrained in the interior

RECOMMENDED FORMULA: *Bupleurum, Dragon Bone, and Oyster Shell Decoction—Chai Hu Jia Long Gu Mu Li Tang*

Chai hu	Rx Bupleuri	12 g
Huang qin	Rx Scutellaria	5 g
Ban xia	Rz Pinellia ternata	6–10 g
Ren shen	Rx Ginseng	5 g
Sheng jiang	Rz Zingiberis recens	5 g
Gui zhi	Rm Cinnamomi cassia	5 g
Fu ling	Sclerotium poria cocos (fungus)	5 g
Long gu	Os Draconis	5 g
Mu li	Concha ostrea (oyster shell)	5 g

Da huang	Rz Rhei	6 g
Da zao	Fr Jujube	6 pieces
Dai zhe shi	Hematitum (mineral)	5 g

MODIFICATIONS:

For nightmares:

| Long dan cao | Rx Gentiana | add 10 g |
| Xia ku cao | Fl Spica prunella | add 10 g |

When there is no constipation:

| Da huang | Rz Rhei | omit 6 g |

Phlegm symptoms like unclear thinking, foggy head, and desire for stimulants:

Shi chang pu	Rz Acori graminei	add 8 g
Yuan zhi	Rx Polygala	add 10 g
Ren shen	Rx Ginseng	omit 5 g

Severe irritability and insomnia:

| Suan zao ren | Sn Zizyphi spinosa | add 15 g |
| Ye jiao teng | Rx Caulis polygoni multiflori | add 10 g |

Muscle spasms of hands and feet (sometimes of back):

Dan shen	Rx Salvia miltiorrhiza	add 60 g
Tai zi shen	Rx Pseudostellaria	add 10 g
Ren shen	Rx Ginseng	omit 5 g

9. Night Sweats Only

OTHER SYMPTOMS: red face, parched lips, dry stools, dark urine

CHINESE DIAGNOSIS: fire from deficiency due to kidney yin not controlling heart fire and weakness of wei qi

RECOMMENDED FORMULA: *Tang Kui and Six-Yellow Decoction— Dong Quai Liu Huang Tang*

Dong quai	Rx Angelica sinensis	10–15 g
Sheng di huang	Rx Rehmannia glutinosa	10–15 g
Huang lian	Rz Coptidis	3–6 g
Huang qin	Rx Scutellaria	6–12 g
Huang bai	Cx Phellodendri	6–15 g
Huang qi	Rx Astragali membranacei	30 g

MODIFICATIONS:
Severe sweating:

| Zhi mu | Rx Anemarrhena | add 10 g |
| Fu xiao mai | Sn Tritici levis | add 10–20 g |

10. Mild Hot Flashes and Night Sweats

OTHER SYMPTOMS: fatigue, sore or weak lower back, diminished hearing, light-headedness, forgetfulness, difficulty concentrating, dry eyes with diminished acuity of vision, prone to joint injuries

CHINESE DIAGNOSIS: kidney and liver yin deficiency

RECOMMENDED FORMULA: *Six-Ingredient Pill with Rehmannia— Liu Wei Di Huang Wan*

Shu di huang	Rx Rehmannia glutinosa	20 g
Shan zhu yu	Fr Corni	10 g
Shan yao	Rx Dioscorea	10 g
Fu ling	Sclerotium poria cocos (fungus)	8 g
Mu dan pi	Cx Moutan radicis	8 g
Ze xie	Rz Alismatis	8 g

MODIFICATIONS:

Severe fluid depletion:

Shu di huang	Rx Rehmannia glutinosa	omit 20 g
Sheng di huang	Rx Rehmannia glutinosa	add 20 g

Rapid weight loss after onset of menopause:

Tian hua fen	Rx Trichosanthis	add 12 g
Ze xie	Rz Alismatis	omit 8 g

Dry eyes, diminished visual acuity, tearing when exposed to wind:

Gou qi zi	Fr Lycii	add 10–15 g
Ju hua	Fl Chrysanthemi	add 10 g

More severe night sweats and hot flashes:

Zhi mu	Rx Anemarrhena	add 10–15 g
Huang bai	Cx Phellodendri	add 10 g

Consumptive dry cough (when taking beta-blockers for hypertension):

Mai men dong	Rx Ophiopogonis	add 10 g
Wu wei zi	Fr Schizandra	add 10 g

11. Hot Flashes That Are Worse in Early Afternoon, with a Sense of Exhaustion (Need of a Nap) or Hot Sensation from Inside the Body While the Exterior Feels Normal

OTHER SYMPTOMS: lethargy, insomnia, night sweats, irritability, emaciation

CHINESE DIAGNOSIS: liver and kidney yin deficiency

RECOMMENDED FORMULA: *Cool the Bones Powder—Qing Gu San*

Yin chai hu	Rx Stellaria dichotoma	10–15 g
Zhi mu	Rx Anemarrhena	10–15 g
Hu huang lian	Rz Picrorrhiza	10 g
Di gu pi	Cx Lycii radicis	10 g
Qin jiao	Rx Gentiana	6 g
Qing hao	Hb Artemisia annua	6 g
Zhi bie jia	Carapax amydae, honey-fried (shell)	10–15 g
Gan cao	Rx Glycyrrhiza uralensis	4 g

MODIFICATIONS:
Pale complexion and low voice:

Huang qi   Rx Astragali membranacei   add 10–20 g

Severe sweats:

Fu xiao mai   Fr Tritici levis   add 10–20 g

More severe tidal fever in afternoon:

Hei dou   Sn Glycine soja   add 10–20 g

12. Hot Flashes and Night Sweats That Are Mild and Appear All Day and Night. May Be More Severe in the Early Morning. Sweating Is Mainly in the Face, Palms, and Feet. May Be Hot

OTHER SYMPTOMS: dry mouth and throat, thirst with a desire to drink, lower back soreness, eye distress, frequent hunger that cannot be satisfied

CHINESE DIAGNOSIS: kidney yin deficiency with essence and marrow depletion

RECOMMENDED FORMULA: *Restore the Left (Kidney) Decoction— Jia Wei Zou Gui Yin*

Shu di huang	Rx Rehmannia glutinosa	15 g
Shan yao	Rx Dioscorea	15 g

Gou qi zi	Fr Lycii	18 g
Shan zhu yu	Fr Corni	12 g
Fu ling	Sclerotium poria cocos (fungus)	12 g
Zhi gan cao	Rx Glycyrrhiza uralensis, honey-fried	6 g
Long gu	Os Draconis	30 g
Mu li	Concha ostrea (oyster shell)	30 g
Bai shao	Rx Paeonia lactiflora	15 g

MODIFICATIONS:

Profuse uterine bleeding:

Han lian cao	Hb Eclipta	add 18 g
Nu zhen zi	Fr Ligustri lucidi	add 15 g
Di yu	Rx Sanguisorba	add 30 g

Breakthrough continuous uterine bleeding with clots:

| Yi mu cao | Hb Leonuri | add 30 g |
| Qian cao gen | Rx Rubiae | add 12 g |

More severe dry mouth and headaches:

Sheng di huang	Rx Rehmannia glutinosa	add 15 g
Shu di huang	Rx Rehmannia glutinosa	omit 15 g
Ju hua	Fl Chrysanthemi	add 10 g
Xia ku cao	Fl Spica prunella	add 12 g
Zhen zhu mu	Concha margarita usta (shell)	add 30 g

Emotional restlessness:

| Fu xiao mai | Fr Tritici levis | add 30 g |
| Zhi gan cao | Rx Glycyrrhiza uralensis, honey-fried | increase to 12 g |

Da zao   Fr Jujube   7 pieces
Shi chang pu Cx Albizia   add 15 g

Profuse spontaneous sweating:

Huang qi   Rx Astragali membranacei   add 30 g
Fu xiao mai   Fr Tritici levis   add 15 g

Severe night sweats:

Wu wei zi   Fr Schizandra   add 15 g

Irritability and early morning hot flashes, sweats, and waking:

Mai men dong   Rx Ophiopogonis   add 12 g

Vaginal dryness:

Huai niu xi   Rx Achyranthis   add 15 g
Shan dou gen   Rx Sophora subprostrata   add 20 g

Bloating, flatulence with spleen qi deficiency:

Sha ren   Fr Amomi   add 10 g
Chen pi   Per Citri reticulata add 10 g

13. Hot Flashes Followed by Cold Sweats and Cold Extremities

OTHER SYMPTOMS: mild sweating throughout the day, especially in area of the upper lip; general edema; loose stools; abdominal distention; night urination; urinary incontinence; lower back and knee weakness, pain, and stiffness

CHINESE DIAGNOSIS: kidney yang deficiency with waning of mingmen fire

RECOMMENDED FORMULA: *Restore the Right (Kidney) Pill—You Gui Wan*

Fu zi	Rx Aconiti carmichaeli	10 g
Rou gui	Cx Cinnamomi	8 g
Lu jiao jiao	Colla cornu cervi (deer-horn gelatin)	12 g
Shu di huang	Rx Rehmannia glutinosa	30 g
Shan zhu yu	Fr Corni	10 g
Shan yao	Rx Dioscorea	12 g
Gou qi zi	Fr Lycii	15 g
Tu si zi	Sn Cuscuta	10 g
Du zhong	Cx Eucommia	10 g
Dong quai	Rx Angelica sinensis	8 g

MODIFICATIONS:

Severe nocturia and urinary incontinence:

Yi zhi ren	Fr Alpinia oxyphylla	add 30 g
Hai piao xiao	Os Sepia seu sepiella	add 15 g
Fu pen zi	Fr Rubi	add 15 g

More severe edema and facial swelling:

Che qian zi	Sn Plantaginis	add 12 g
Ze xie	Rz Alismatis	add 10 g

Decreased libido:

Yin yang huo	Hb Epimedi	add 30 g
Xian mao	Rz Curculiginis orchioidis	add 15 g

Diarrhea:

Gan jiang	Rz Zingiberis	add 6 g
Lian zi xin	Fl Plumula nelumbinis	add 12 g
Chi shi zhi	Halloysitum rubrum (crimson stone resin)	add 15 g
Rou dou kou	Sn Myristica	add 15 g

For more severe cold, painful feet:

Bu gu zhi   Fr Psoralea   add 10 g

For abdominal pain:

Wu zhu yu   Fr Evodia   add 15 g

14. Low-Grade Hot Flash and Mild Sweat in Face and Chest All Day Long

OTHER SYMPTOMS: dark complexion; soreness in waist, hip, and knees; alternating discomfort of hot and cold extremities with a sense of weakness in limbs and mild numbness; decreased libido

CHINESE DIAGNOSIS: kidney yin and yang deficiency

RECOMMENDED FORMULA: *Modified Decoction of Curculigo and Epimedi with Pill of Glossy Privet Fruit and Eclipta*

Yin yang huo	Hb Epimedi	10 g
Xian mao	Rz Curculiginis orchioidis	10 g
Ba ji tian	Rx Morinda officinalis	10 g
Nu zhen zi	Fr Ligustri lucidi	10 g
Han lian cao	Hb Eclipta	10 g
Shu di huang	Rx Rehmannia glutinosa	10 g
Dong quai	Rx Angelica sinensis	10 g
Zhi mu	Rx Anemarrhena	10 g
Huang bai	Cx Phellodendri	10 g

15. Sweating Without Much Heat Around Neck or Above the Lips

OTHER SYMPTOMS: anxiety, dry skin, dry hair and mouth, itching, constipation

CHINESE DIAGNOSIS: kidney yin deficiency without much deficient heat

RECOMMENDED FORMULA: *Empirical Prescription Dr. Chun*

Sheng di huang	Rx Rehmannia glutinosa	6 g
Shu di huang	Rx Rehmannia glutinosa	6 g
Gui ban	Plastrum testudinis (freshwater turtle shell)	12 g
Mu li	Concha ostrea (oyster shell)	12 g
Gou teng	Rm Uncaria	6 g
Suan zao ren	Sn Zizyphi spinosa	5 g
Fu ling	Sclerotium poria cocos (fungus)	6 g
Fu shen	Poria cocos pararadicis (fungus)	6 g

16. Hot Flashes and Night Sweats That Are Triggered Mainly by Emotional Reactions of Any Kind, Including Dreams

OTHER SYMPTOMS: Mental restlessness, light-headedness or heavy-headedness

CHINESE DIAGNOSIS: kidney yin deficiency with deficient heart and liver fire

RECOMMENDED FORMULA: *Menopause Formula—Geng Nian Fang*

Sheng di huang	Rx Rehmannia glutinosa	10 g
Nu zhen zi	Fr Ligustri lucidi	6 g
Han lian cao	Hb Eclipta	5 g
Suan zao ren	Sn Zizyphi spinosa	5 g
Long chi	Dens draconis (fossilized mammal teeth)	12 g

Gou teng	Rm Uncaria	6 g
Lian zi xin	Fl Plumula nelumbinis	5 g
Fu ling	Sclerotium poria cocos (fungus)	6 g
He huan pi	Cx Albizia	6 g
Zi cao	Rx Lithospermi	5 g

17. Hot Flashes Without Much Sweating, Accompanied by Sensation of Cold Feet, Exhaustion, and Dry Throat

CHINESE DIAGNOSIS: primarily kidney yin and mild yang deficiency
RECOMMENDED FORMULA: *Peaceful Menopause—Geng Nian An*

Shu di huang	Rx Rehmannia glutinosa	10 g
Ze xie	Rz Alismatis	6 g
Fu ling	Sclerotium poria cocos (fungus)	6 g
Mu dan pi	Cx Moutan radicis	6 g
Shan yao	Rx Dioscorea	6 g
Shan zhu yu	Fr Corni	6 g
Sheng di huang	Rx Rehmannia glutinosa	6 g
He shou wu	Rx Polygoni multiflori	6 g
Xian mao	Rz Curculiginis orchioidis	6 g

MODIFICATIONS:
Itching:

Chan tui	Periostracum cicadae (cicada moulting)	6 g
Fang feng	Rx Ledebouriella	6 g
Hai tong pi	Cx Erythrinia	4 g
Yu zhu	Rx Polygonati odorati	8 g

Dizziness and headache:

Tian ma	Rx Gastrodia	6 g
Gou teng	Rm Uncaria	6 g
Shi jue ming	Concha haliotidis (abalone shell)	10 g

| Niu xi | Rx Achyranthis | 8 g |
| Sang ji sheng | Rm Loranthi seu visci | 10 g |

18. Mild Hot Flashes Throughout the Day That Seem to Come and Go

OTHER SYMPTOMS: premature menopause (stopping of menses) from late thirties to mid-forties; menopausal symptoms experienced mostly emotional

CHINESE DIAGNOSIS: depression of heart, liver, and spleen qi blocking the menses

RECOMMENDED FORMULA: *Boost the Menses Decoction— Yi Jing Tang*

Shu di huang	Rx Rehmannia glutinosa	30 g
Bai zhu	Rx Atractylodes macrocephala	30 g
Shan yao	Rx Dioscorea	15 g
Dong quai	Rx Angelica sinensis	15 g
Bai shao	Rx Paeonia lactiflora	10 g
Suan zao ren	Sn Zizyphi spinosa	10 g
Mu dan pi	Cx Moutan radicis	6 g
Bei sha shen	Rx Glehnia	10 g
Chai hu	Rx Bupleuri	3 g
Du zhong	Cx Eucommia	3 g
Ren shen	Rx Ginseng	6 g

19. Hot Flashes and Night Sweats

OTHER SYMPTOMS: irregular onset of menses and irregular amount of menstrual flow, dizziness, vertigo, lumbar pain, cold limbs, lack of strength, bland taste in mouth, edema, loose stools, night urination

CHINESE DIAGNOSIS: kidney and spleen deficiency in perimenopause

RECOMMENDED FORMULA: *Menopause Formula Dr. Liu*

| Shan yao | Rx Dioscorea | 10 g |
| Lian zi | Sn Nelumbinis | 10 g |

Tu si zi	Sn Cuscuta	8 g
Xu duan	Rx Dipsaci	8 g
Shu di huang	Rx Rehmannia glutinosa	12 g
Fu pen zi	Fr Rubi	10 g
Bai zhu	Rx Atractylodes macrocephala	8 g
Fu ling	Sclerotium poria cocos (fungus)	10 g
Yin yang huo	Hb Epimedi	8 g
Xian mao	Rz Curculiginis orchioidis	8 g

MODIFICATIONS:

More spleen deficiency with whole body edema and continuous spotting:
Gui pi tang—restore-the-spleen decoction with Fang feng (Rx Sileris) and Qiang huo (Rx Notopterigii)

Heavy bleeding:

Huang qi	Rx Astragali membranacei	add 12 g
Zong lu	Fibra stipula trachycarpi (palm stipule)	add 8 g
Ce bai ye	Cacumen biota (leafy twigs)	add 8 g
E jiao	Gelatinum corii asini (donkey-hide gelatin)	add 10 g

20. Hot Flashes at Night and Night Sweats in Lower Back Area

OTHER SYMPTOMS: weak voice, low appetite, dry throat, irregular menses with diminished flow

CHINESE DIAGNOSIS: spleen qi deficiency with kidney yang deficiency and kidney and liver yin deficiency

RECOMMENDED FORMULA: *Old Buddha's Vital Energy-Building and Yin-Reinforcing Syrup—Lao Fo Ye Fu Yuan Yi Gao*

Dang shen	Rx Codonopsis	30 g
Bai zhu	Rx Atractylodes macrocephala	30 g
Fu ling	Sclerotium poria cocos (fungus)	30 g
Bai shao	Rx Paeonia lactiflora	30 g
Dong quai	Rx Angelica sinensis	30 g

Di gu pi	Cx Lycii radicis	30 g
Mu dan pi	Cx Moutan radicis	18 g
Sha ren	Fr Amomi	12 g
Yin chai hu	Rx Stellaria dichotoma	10 g
Zi su ye	Fl Perilla	3 g
Bo he	Hb Mentha	3 g
Lu jiao jiao	Colla cornu cervi (deer-horn gelatin)	15 g
Xiang fu	Rz Cyperi rotundi	18 g

Treating Insomnia

Anyone who has experienced insomnia will recognize this vicious cycle: You can't sleep, so you're tired during the day. You're tired, so you crave stimulants like caffeine and sweets. After drinking caffeine and eating sweets, you can't sleep, so you take medicine to help you sleep. But the medicine makes you feel drowsy the next day, so you drink lots of coffee and eat too many sweets again.

On top of this, you are afraid of becoming addicted to the drugs, which makes you feel stressed out and confused. You turn to chamomile tea and valerian root to calm your nerves, and you weigh the pros and cons of taking melatonin. You try drinking a glass of warm milk or a shot of liquor before bed, none of which works. You're simply exhausted.

Most drugs prescribed for insomnia are good for putting you to sleep but are not good at making sure that you don't wake up throughout the night. The herbs we prescribe for sleep during menopause are for making sure you stay sleeping throughout the night and not just to "knock" you into sleep.

In traditional Chinese medicine, there are herbs that are helpful in treating what we call "deficiency-induced sleep disorders." The point is to induce relaxation and natural sleep, not drug a patient into an unnatural and, ultimately, unsatisfying sleep cycle. Listed below are herbs and minerals I recommend for insomnia, and herbs I suggest you stay away from if you have trouble sleeping. The recommended substances should be taken as part of a comprehensive formula or a specific formula for sleep.

HERBS AND MINERALS FOR INSOMNIA	HERBS TO AVOID WITH INSOMNIA
Zizyphus seed *Suan zao ren*	Processed Aconite root *Fu zi*
Schizandra fruit *Wu wei zi*	Ginseng root *Ren shen* (at night)
Biota seed *Bai zi ren*	Aurantium fruit *Zhi shi*
Oyster shell *Mu li*	Lonicera flower *Jin yin hua*
Polygoni multiflori stem *Ye jiao teng*	

Treating Sexual Dysfunction

Many women complain of diminished libido after the onset of menopause. This is not because women just "don't like it" anymore, but the result of actual physiological changes that come with the natural decline of your reproductive hormones. With the decline of hormones often come vaginal dryness and vaginal atrophy, which make sexual arousal and intercourse difficult and sometimes painful.

Sexuality has occupied the minds of Chinese physicians for centuries, and there are libraries full of manuals and detailed treatment strategies on the subject. Traditional Chinese practitioners are taught that the question of sexuality is one of the ten essential questions for diagnosis of any internal disorder. Sexual function isn't thought of in psychological terms; it is thought of in terms of the relationship of the body's amount of available energy and the way this resource is distributed. Health is not measured just by being robust but also by evenly utilizing one's energy resources. So, as we discussed before, during menopause the body goes into preservation mode in order to protect vital functions. Since sexuality is closely related to reproduction, it will take time until the change is complete and reorganized.

In traditional Chinese medicine, we divide decreased libido into four aspects and treat each individually, as necessary: (1) lack of mental desire, (2) lack of physical arousal, (3) mechanical difficulty or inability, and (4) relationship problems.

Traditional Chinese medicine has herbs for the first three problems—for the fourth, we offer simple advice. For example, it is thought that the herb yin yang huo (*Epimedium grandiflorum*) increases libido and that the formula Rehmannia Eight (Ba Wei Di Huang Wan) increases the production of testosterone that may increase the libido.

Vaginal dryness is often treated with the combination of herbs that increase moisture, those that lower inflammation, and those that promote tissue growth. Examples are Zhi mu (*Anemarrhena asphodeloides*) for moisture, Ku shen (*Sophora flavecentis*) for inflammation, and Xiang fu (*Cyperus rotundus*) for tissue formation. The herbs can be used internally as well as intravaginally. Addressing all three problems generally resolves the dryness, atrophy, and pain as one problem rather than separately.

As for the advice: It isn't unusual for couples to go through difficult times during the woman's menopause, which is often accompanied by sexual confusion—for the man as well as the woman. The best advice I can give is not to give up on sex, to communicate the best you can, and to be patient with yourself and your partner. In Chinese medicine, sexual play is considered important for one's health and well-being. We believe sex helps maintain a healthy relationship between the mind and the vital organs, which Chinese medicine believes will result in greater health and graceful aging.

Treating and Preventing Osteoporosis

Women often come to my practice bearing bone mineral density (BMD) scans that indicate they are either osteoporotic or osteopenic, meaning they have significant bone loss or are on their way to having significant bone loss. Their doctors have offered them drugs like Fosamax or Evista, both of which are effective at slowing down bone loss but have undesirable long-term side effects. (Fosamax can cause erosion of the esophagus, and Evista may cause hot flashes and blood clots.) These women are often nervous and confused about their options—or seeming lack of options.

When it comes to Western medicine the options are: Suffer continued bone loss or take the drugs and live with the side effects. But there are other alternatives. Chinese medicine offers many remedies and techniques that can help. There is one catch, though—changes in bone density typically don't show up on a scan until after at least one year of treatment. This can be frustrating for Western medical doctors and the women in treatment, since our society is used to the idea that there is a "magic pill" that will treat whatever ails them—fast.

A few years ago, a seventy-eight-year-old woman who I had seen on and off for various reasons over many years came to see me. She had been given a diagnosis of osteoporosis. She was generally not inclined to take any pharmaceutical drugs. But on the rare occasions she did, she carefully researched the medication before taking it—weighing the risks and benefits. She was not comfortable with the drug she had been prescribed, or the side effects she read about, but her doctor had offered her no other choices. She had taken the prescription with her but then decided to consult me before actually filling it.

I prescribed an herbal formula for her, which she took daily for one year. After a year, she went to her doctor for another bone scan. When she called for her results a week later, the nurse got on the phone and said the doctor wanted to talk to her. In a jovial voice, he asked how she liked the new pill he'd prescribed. Had she experienced any side effects yet? He was amazed at its effectiveness—*after only a year, she had the bones of a twenty-year-old.* She's had three bone scans since she's been taking the herbs, and her osteoporosis has not returned.

Osteoporosis occurs when the body fails to form enough new bone or when too much old bone is reabsorbed by the body. It is a bone-thinning disease characterized by a loss of bone mass and deterioration in bone structure. This leads to an increased risk of bone fracture, particularly of the spine, hip, and wrist. The single most important thing you can do to prevent osteoporosis and maintain your bone strength is to exercise. Get your heart, lungs, and muscles working, and your body will activate its own healing capacity.

The herbs most often prescribed for women with osteoporosis or osteopenia are listed in the table below.

PROMOTE BONE CALCIFICATION	PROMOTE HEALING OF FRACTURES	CONTAIN PHYTOESTROGENS	PROVEN TO WORK IN CLINICAL TRIALS
Psorala fruit *Bu gu zhi*	Deer horn *Lu rong*	Psorala fruit *Bu gu zhi*	Modified Rehmannia Six *Liu wei di huang wan*
Drynaria root *Gu sui bu*	Sarcandra herb *Jiu jie feng*	Cyperi tuber *Xiang fu*	Kidney-nourishing and bone-strengthening pill

Treating Memory Loss and Other Cognitive Dysfunctions

As they age, many women experience diminished cognitive functions in areas such as short-term memory, multitasking, calculation ability, and coming up with words when speaking or writing. Loss of cognitive function often occurs slowly, first only slightly affecting short-term memory. Later it may affect your ability to do simple things like add numbers or find the right words. Soon everyday tasks can become a challenge. For example, you might pick up your keys, put on your coat, and forget where you're going. Of course, all of us have had those moments when we can't find our glasses or we forget someone's name. The difference in this case is that for some menopausal women these "moments" become more and more frequent and start to have a significant effect on their lives.

In Chinese medicine, we prescribe various herbs to increase cognitive functioning such as memory. *Evodia rutaecarpa* (wu zhu yu) and *Polygala tenuifolia* (yuan zhi) are examples of herbs that support mental function. There are several clinical trials from Hong Kong, Japan, and China that looked at treating senile dementia with herbs such as alpinia oxyphylla fruit (yi zhi), evodia fruit (wu zhu yu), and salvia root (dan shen), as well as with acupuncture. The studies suggest that herbs and acupuncture can benefit the cognitive function of the elderly. All the trials showed increases in daily functioning, ability to read, and participation in family activities.

There is even one Western drug (Huperizine-A), which is derived from an old Chinese herb, that is currently being developed under the FDA guidelines for the treatment of Alzheimer's disease and senile dementia.

The Future of Menopause Treatment

Important changes—in metabolism, immunity, skin condition, and cognitive function—occur during menopause. They are considered to be directly and indirectly related to the decline in reproductive ability and to the effects reproductive hormones such as estrogen have on nonreproductive tissues. We now know definitively that there is a correlation between these changes and the reproductive hormones. However, estrogen is not just a reproductive hormone; its effect on the body is far more global.

There are many treatments that were used in the past by Chinese physicians that can guide us in developing future menopause treatments. Concepts such as qi and essence, yin and yang must be translated into scientific language like receptors and transcription, genes and proteins in order to study their effects scientifically.

I have been working on doing this for eight years in an attempt to find new, safer, and more precise treatment for women going through menopause. My colleagues Dale Leitman and Mary Tagliaferri and I, at UCSF and Bionovo, Inc., have studied the physiology of menopause and the molecular mechanisms underlying it. We have discovered that what Western medicine has come up with to treat menopause—primarily hormone replacement—brings with it significant risk of developing illnesses such as heart disease, breast cancer, and stroke.

We have started to use genomic and molecular tools to describe and potentially profile the risks associated with using hormones for individual women. For instance, the risk of getting breast cancer from the use of HRT is very small (eight additional cases above normal for every ten thousand women using HRT for one year). Yet we cannot identify in advance who these women might be. If we can profile this risk, it will allow us to exclude these women from ever being exposed to this risk. We have also been testing and manipulating herbal formulas in an attempt to create therapies from traditional herbs—that have been used safely and effectively for centuries—to manage and treat many symptoms of menopause such as hot flashes, osteoporosis, and reduced cognitive function.

In fact, we have just recently completed a clinical trial for the first of these drugs. We are now entering the next stage, which will include two or three more placebo-controlled trials before these therapies will be available to the public. I believe that in the next decade we will have not one but a variety of herbal treatment options for menopausal women that are proven safe, specific, and effective under the blessing of an FDA approval process.

5 Phytoestrogens and Natural Hormones

Tori Hudson, N.D.

Tori Hudson has been teaching and in clinical practice for twenty years. She is currently a professor at the National College of Naturopathic Medicine and Bastyr University in Seattle, and medical director at A Woman's Time in Portland, Oregon. Dr. Hudson was named Physician of the Year in 1999 by the American Association of Naturopathic Physicians, has been a consultant to the National Institutes of Health and the natural products industry, serves on many advisory panels, and is a nationally known speaker and author. She is the author of the acclaimed herbal medicine book Women's Encyclopedia of Natural Medicine *(Keats Publishing, 1999).*

Many perimenopausal and postmenopausal women come to me because they are not satisfied with the treatment options offered to them by their doctors and are looking for alternative ways to treat their menopausal symptoms. Unfortunately, when women reach menopause, they are frequently presented with only two options: take some form of replacement hormone therapy or live with significant symptoms and risk osteoporosis. For most women, however, there are other choices.

Naturopathic medicine incorporates many therapeutic modalities: herbal medicine, homeopathy, nutrition, nutraceuticals, hydrotherapy, exercise therapy, physical therapy, bodywork, and lifestyle and psychological counseling. I utilize all of these as well as conventional medical approaches in my practice.

But how do you make the decision? There are so many conflicting points of view. The important thing to remember is that no two women's menopausal transitions are alike, and each woman responds differently to treatment methods. This means that while conventional HRT may work for lots of women with no side effects, it might not work for you—and the same is true for natural remedies. Fortunately for women, today there are many choices for treating symptoms of menopause.

Women who don't want to take hormones, and those who cannot for a variety of reasons, such as a history of breast cancer or heart disease, can manage their health and well-being with a variety of natural therapies such as herbs and botanicals, vitamins and nutritional supplements, healthy food, and exercise. Options such as these have been shown to relieve some of the worst symptoms of menopause, including menstrual irregularities, hot flashes, night sweats, vaginal dryness, fatigue, decreased libido, mood swings, weight gain, depression, anxiety, changes in memory and cognition, sleep disturbance, nausea, headaches, and urinary incontinence (for more on managing this and other bladder problems, see chapter 8).

You can find a complete discussion of natural therapies that are used to treat menopausal symptoms throughout this book. In this chapter, I focus on two increasingly important aspects of naturopathic medicine in the treatment of menopause: phytoestrogens, compounds found in plants that have estrogenlike properties; and natural hormones, hormones that are biochemically identical to human hormones and are made in a laboratory from compounds extracted from plants.

Today's health-care providers—whether medical doctors or alternative practitioners—are increasingly willing to work with you to evaluate and manage your symptoms on an individual basis, as opposed to simply prescribing a standard medical regimen. Working with your practitioner, you can request information, educate yourself, and take charge of your treatment options. When deciding on a course of treatment with your health-care provider, keep in mind that some of these common symptoms could be products of the normal aging process or life circumstances and not directly related to the hormonal fluctuations of menopause.

Phytoestrogens: Plants with Estrogenlike Qualities

The old adage "Eat your vegetables" is especially true for women in menopause; more than three hundred plants contain phytoestrogens, a naturally occurring plant hormone. Phytoestrogens are a group of chemicals found in plants that can act like the hormone estrogen. Phytoestrogens may affect the production and/or breakdown of estrogen by the body as well as the levels of estrogen carried in the bloodstream. Estrogen is necessary for childbearing and can have a variety of effects on different organ systems. Most food phytoestrogens are from three chemical classes—isoflavones, lignans, and coumestans.

SOY ISOFLAVONES

Isoflavones are found in beans from the legume family; soybeans and other soy-based products are the major dietary source of this type of phytoestrogen. Women in perimenopause and menopause have become increasingly interested in isoflavones, as they have a similar structure to the sex hormones that are naturally present in the body. They bind to estrogen receptors on human cells, and as a result, they have weaker but similar effects on the central nervous system, blood vessels, and bone and skin, as compared with a woman's premenopausal hormones. Isoflavones may be able to do this without stimulating the breast or uterus, which could minimize any risk for developing breast or uterine cancer, two risks that are associated with hormone replacement therapy.[1]

There is much controversy about the effects of soy on breasts. Perhaps the most comprehensive scientific review of the topic can be found in an important article published in 2001. After a review of 270 published scientific papers on the topic, and a consideration of laboratory, animal, and human research, the conclusion is that for breast cancer survivors, a serving of soy on a daily basis is probably safe.[2] The benefit of soy for premenopausal and postmenopausal women (without breast cancer) is inconsistent.

While eating soybeans and other soy products (such as tofu, tempeh, and soy milk) is a healthy way to get isoflavones into your diet, realistically there is no way to eat enough soy products to produce the effects of HRT. There are a number of dietary supplements that contain large quantities of isoflavones, and some of these may be used for hot flashes and bone health; 50–150 mg of soy isoflavones are doses that may offer some therapeutic benefit. It is estimated that soy isoflavones have only 1/400 to 1/1,000 the potency of estradiol—the principal estrogen secreted by the ovaries in premenopausal women. So while isoflavones can definitely mimic some of the effects of estrogen, they are not likely to be a magic pill for menopausal symptoms.

There are also potential side effects of eating too many soybeans, although I consider these to be rare. One area of concern for some is the phytate content in soybeans. Phytates can block the uptake of minerals such as calcium, magnesium, iron, and zinc. However, if you eat soy products in the context of a healthy, varied diet, you should get adequate minerals. The genestein and daidzein in soy can also inhibit thyroid hormone synthesis. High-soybean diets have been implicated in diet-induced goiter. However, this occurred long ago, when children were fed iodine-deficient soy infant formula; once iodine was added to the infant formulations, this adverse effect was mitigated. The problem is not likely to occur if you are eating an average amount of soy. In addition, soy foods, especially cooked soybeans, are difficult for some people to digest, causing gas and stomach upset.

That said, some studies suggest that reasonably increasing soy foods in your diet can help regulate the menstrual cycle,[3] stabilize bone density,[4] reduce cholesterol,[5] and lessen some symptoms of menopause. One of the most recent studies of soy and menopausal symptoms demonstrated positive results. The change in menopausal symptoms and cardiovascular risk factors was evaluated when eighty women were randomized in a double-blind, placebo-controlled study. Forty women were given 10 mg of soy isoflavones, and forty women were given a placebo for four months. In the first follow-up visit at one month, symptoms were similar between the two groups. During the full four-month treatment period, though, the menopausal symptoms of the women using soy isoflavones were significantly lower than those of the women who received a placebo. The symptoms that improved most included hot flashes and night sweats, insomnia, nervousness, melancholia, vertigo, weakness, and headache. Total cholesterol and LDL (risk factors for heart disease) decreased significantly in the isoflavone group compared with levels pre-treatment or in the placebo group.[6]

Most of the research on soy isoflavones, however, has been done on symptoms like hot flashes and night sweats, and results have been mixed. The mixed results of the studies on soy to date can be in part attributed to the fact that the studies varied in the form of the soy product that was tested—for example, some studies used soy foods, while others used isolated soy isoflavones or soy protein without isoflavones. So, despite some promising results, it's not possible to say with certainty which form of soy is the most effective in treating menopausal symptoms. However, having 50 to 150 mg of soy isoflavones in the diet is a reasonable approach.

LIGNANS

Lignans are found in high-fiber foods such as cereal brans and beans; flaxseeds also contain large amounts. Lignans are weaker than soy phytoestrogens—meaning they may have fewer negative effects, but they have fewer positive ones as well. However, the accumulation of phytoestrogens from flaxseeds may have other health benefits: providing additional fiber, possibly reducing the risk of osteoporosis and breast cancer, possibly improving lipid profiles, and favorably altering the body's metabolism of estrogen. Ground flaxseeds are an easy way to add lignans to your diet; they can be combined with cereal, smoothies, yogurt, rice, or soy milk, or baked into muffins.

COUMESTANS

Coumestans are found in various beans such as pinto beans and lima beans, as well as split peas; alfalfa and clover sprouts are the foods with the highest amounts of coumestans.

Red clover (*Trifolium pratense*), which contains coumestan, is a member of the legume family and is rich in flavonoids, glycosides, phytoestrogens, and other vitamins and minerals. This Native American herb was traditionally used to treat whooping cough, gout, and cancer. Today, it has gained popularity as a treatment for menopausal symptoms. Eating foods high in coumestans may have a modest effect on relieving hot flashes and night sweats. There have been several clinical trials that have studied the effect of red clover phytoestrogens on symptoms of menopause such as hot flashes and night sweats, but the results have been mixed. The ideal dose of red clover isoflavones is 50 mg of standardized extract twice a day (for more on red clover, see chapter 3).

Natural Hormones Versus Synthetic Hormones

One of the greatest areas of confusion in natural medicine today is the subject of natural hormones versus other hormones. Natural hormones, commonly called "bio-identical" hormones (compounded estrogens, progesterone, testosterone, dehydroepiandrosterone [DHEA], and natural progesterone creams), are distinct from conjugated equine estrogens, conjugated plant estrogens, synthetic estrogens, and synthetic progestins in that they have a molecular structure identical to the natural hormones made by the body. By contrast, synthetic hormones are intentionally different in chemical makeup from the body's natural hormones. There are also hormones made from a natural substance that are not bio-identical.

The most well known example of this is Premarin, made from more than two hundred compounds found in the urine of pregant mares. Because drug companies cannot patent a natural structure, they invent hormones that are patentable (such as Premarin, Prempro, and Provera).

For the past sixty years, conjugated equine estrogen, brand-name Premarin, has been the most commonly prescribed estrogen supplement in the United States. Synthetic estrogens are man-made estrogens that are also not bio-identical.

There are now several branded versions of natural hormones that are available for hormone replacement therapy.

It is the *chemical structure* of a hormone, not its *source,* that determines if a hormone is natural or synthetic. A natural hormone can be developed in a laboratory using pharmaceutical-grade products. Natural hormones are most often made from phytoestrogens extracted from soybeans or Mexican wild yam root. The extracted compounds are made in a laboratory into hormones that are identical to the hormone your body naturally produces.

There are several possible benefits to using natural hormones over synthetic hormones. First, natural hormones are thought to be metabolized more favorably by your body than the synthetic types. Second, with natural hormones, health-care providers can create customized dosing regimens and potencies to fit each individual woman, which can then be adjusted in small units to taper someone on to or off of treatment. Third, a natural hormone such as natural progesterone may have a friendlier effect on the breast and cardiovascular systems. Fourth, natural hormones can have reduced side effects, especially in the case of progesterone.

Natural hormones also have a much shorter half-life—meaning, they take less time to be eliminated from your body by natural processes. Last, other types of hormone treatments may have additives, binders, or preservatives included in their formulations.

I am not suggesting that bio-identical hormones are innately good and non-bio-identical hormones are innately bad. Much of the decision as to which kind of hormone to take depends on the woman. Some women can't take the non-bio-identical version because of past medical problems, or don't want to because of the side effects—severe bloating, mood swings, and irritability, for example—or because they want a more natural approach.

Theoretically, a dose of natural hormone that is equivalent in strength to a dose of other hormone (used in HRT) should produce the same benefits. However, there has not been enough research done to date to determine this definitively. Some would argue that the advantage of conventional HRT is that it has undergone years of scientific study. While this is true, many of the results have been inconsistent, and some have shown that HRT increases the risk of certain serious illnesses (for more on this, see chapter 2). Although there has been relatively little scientific study to date on the safety and efficacy of natural hormones to treat menopause, in my practice I tend to recommend natural hormones almost exclusively. The ability to individualize prescriptions and to provide endless options and flexibility is invaluable. Also, as you will see, combining estriol with estradiol and/or using natural progesterone provides the potential maximum benefit, with *possibly* less risk than conventional hormones.

Natural Estrogen Therapy

Estrogen is the major hormone that has been used to treat menopausal symptoms. There are three dominant estrogens in the body: estradiol, estrone, and estriol. Estradiol is the primary estrogen produced by the ovaries. Estrone is formed from estradiol. Estriol is produced in large amounts during pregnancy and is a breakdown product of estradiol and estrone. Before menopause, estradiol is the body's predominant estrogen; after menopause, estradiol levels drop so that estrone becomes the predominant estrogen.

Natural estrogen preparations mirror these three naturally occurring estrogens in your body. Health-care providers and pharmacists can prepare formulations of each estrogen alone or in combination with one another, with progesterone, or even with DHEA (dehydroepiandrosterone, a natural steroid hormone produced from cholesterol by the adrenal glands) and testosterone. The ability to combine hormones and prescribe varying strengths means that they can be tailored to suit the individual needs of a specific menopausal woman.

All estrogens, natural or otherwise, are prescription medications. Practitioners who use alternative therapies—licensed M.D., D.O., N.P., P.A., or naturopathic physician (N.D.)—can write prescriptions for natural hormones, and then the pharmacists do the *compounding:* putting together various ingredients in specific amounts to create customized medications. There are approximately 1,500 compounding pharmacists in the United States. If there is not a compounding pharmacist in your town or city, a licensed practitioner can write a prescription to one of the many pharmacies that conduct mail-order business.

ESTRIOL

Naturally occurring estriol is produced by the body almost exclusively during pregnancy. It is also formed from the metabolism of estradiol and estriol. Practitioners of alternative medicine use estriol primarily to treat menopausal symptoms because it is considered to be the safest form of estrogen; it is also thought that it might be less carcinogenic than estradiol and estrone.

Several researchers have studied the use of estriol on postmenopausal women. Some of the symptoms that were alleviated with estriol treatment included hot flashes, insomnia, and vaginal dryness and itching during intercourse. A common problem associated with menopause is atrophic vaginitis, a condition that occurs when estrogen is lacking in the body. Symptoms may include vaginal dryness, pain with penetration, increased frequency of vaginal and urinary tract infections, urinary incontinence, and urinary frequency and urgency.

Estriol can be taken orally, in a vaginal tablet, or intravaginally in a cream, gel, or suppository to treat urinary incontinence, urgency, and persistent urinary tract infections. I often prescribe estriol vaginal cream or suppositories for dry or itchy tissue, urinary incontinence, and recurrent urinary tract infections. These creams most likely work by restoring the vaginal flora and increasing lubrication, elasticity, and thickness of the vaginal skin cells. A common prescription is 1 mg of estriol per 1 g of cream. One gram daily for two to four weeks is a good loading dose, and then it is important to decrease to 1 g of cream inserted in the vagina twice a week as a maintenance program (see below).

Estriol: Oral estriol dosing typically ranges from 1 mg/day to 3 mg/day.

Estriol vaginal cream: Estriol 1 mg/g of cream. Insert 1 g every night for two weeks, or twice weekly for eight months.

Estriol and Endometrial Cancer

Although there has been a good deal of study of the effects of estriol therapy on the endometrial or uterine lining (conventional estrogen therapies cause a thickening or overgrowth of the lining, called endometrial hyperplasia, which can lead to cancer), there have been mixed results. In the doses we typically use per day—1 mg, or even up to 3 mg—there appears to be no thickening of the lining of the uterus. If I were prescribing higher doses, then I would advise using estriol along with a proven progestational agent to protect the lining from this thickening effect.

Estriol and Heart Disease Risk

Estriol has not been studied as extensively as conventional HRT in terms of its effect on the risk for heart disease; however, there are a few studies that indicate positive effects of estriol, while others have found estriol to have no effect on blood cholesterol levels, a precursor of heart disease.[7] There is no clear risk or benefit related to estriol and heart disease, compared with the use of estradiol or the common conventional estrogen prescriptions.

Estriol and Bone Density

Estriol also has been minimally studied regarding its effects on bone density and loss; therefore, I do not use estriol to slow or prevent bone loss or to treat low bone density. The research is just not convincing enough at this point. However, estriol taken with calcium supplements may modestly help prevent bone loss that occurs during menopause.

Estriol and Breast Cancer

Women often opt against conventional HRT because they are afraid that it might put them at risk, for breast cancer. Many practitioners and researchers agree that there is a risk, and they have been searching for safer hormone replacement options. This has led some to study and use estriol for treating breast cancer.

Henry Lemon, M.D., a leading researcher on estriol, has concluded that small doses of estriol given in a noncontinuous dosing or cyclic schedule provide protection from breast cancer. Although his hypothesis and work are interesting and offer an appealing basis in which to use estriol, his findings have not been followed up with rigorous clinical trials. The results of other research have not been promising.[8] Estriol, estrone, and estradiol all stimulated human breast cancer cells in tissue cultures. However, estriol may reduce the negative effects of the cancer drug tamoxifen for women already diagnosed with breast cancer.[9]

Prescribing Estriol

So, what does all this mean when it comes to taking estriol or not? Estriol seems to be helpful in treating many of the symptoms of menopause such as hot flashes. However, the jury is still out as to whether estriol will protect you from such conditions as osteoporosis and heart disease. There is some evidence that estriol may provide some benefit to women who are at mild risk for osteoporosis and heart disease or women who are at high risk for breast cancer. Women who currently have breast cancer or who are survivors must weigh the benefits and risks, after being provided with well-balanced information. However, given the current available research, the prudent thing for breast cancer survivors to do is to avoid the use of oral estriol. Vaginal estriol taken to relieve vaginal dryness is considered safe.

A popular practice for prescribing compounded natural estrogens is to combine the potentially safe effects of estriol with small doses of estradiol and estrone, which are thought to help prevent osteoporosis. Currently, those of us who prescribe a tri-estrogen compound to our patients typically use a formula composed of 80 percent estriol, 10 percent estradiol, and 10 percent estrone. Progesterone is added to the formula at a minimum of 50 mg twice a day to protect the uterus from the potential effects of the estrogen in thickening the lining of the endometrium. Using estrogen only, without the proper dose of progesterone, in a patient with a uterus might put her at risk for endometrial hyperplasia (an overgrowth or thickening of the uterine lining) or even endometrial (uterine) cancer.

I also use a bi-estrogen formulation, which is increasingly popular because of concerns that estrone may have a greater role in causing breast cancer than the other two forms of estrogen (estradiol and estriol) that are produced in our bodies. (See below for recommended dose ratios for both tri-estrogen and bi-estrogen formulations.)

> **Tri-estrogen formulation** considered comparable to
> 0.625 mg Premarin/2.5 mg Provera =
> Estriol 1 mg/estradiol 0.125 mg/estrone 0.125 mg/progesterone
> 50 mg, 1 cap twice daily
> **Bi-estrogen formulation** considered equivalent to
> 0.625 mg Premarin/2.5 mg Provera =
> Estriol 1 mg/estradiol 0.250 mg/progesterone 50 mg, 1 cap twice
> daily

Natural Progesterone

Many people mistakenly speak of progesterone when what they really mean is its synthetic counterpart, progestin. *Progesterone* is the term applied to another natural hormone your ovaries make in addition to estrogen, and its main function is to support pregnancy. After menopause, the ovaries stop producing progesterone. *Progestin* is the term applied to the synthetic derivatives, which differ in biochemical structure from progesterone. Progestins are the synthetic hormones used in conventional hormone replacement therapy and birth control pills, and are what often account for the side effects that some women feel when taking these medications, such as irritability, depression, bloating, and mood swings. These side effects are due to progestin's tendency to cause water retention, affect brain chemistry, and alter other steroid pathways. *Progestogen* is a term applied to any substance possessing progesterone qualities. It can refer to progesterone or progestin.

During the perimenopausal phase, when a woman may have months or years of irregular ovulation, her production of progesterone begins to decline. Progesterone falls to almost zero in the beginning of menopause, while estrogen levels decline to only about 40 to 60 percent of premenopausal levels. This progesterone deficiency explains many of the perimenopausal symptoms, such as mood swings, hot flashes, vaginal dryness, and irregular menses.

When estrogen becomes the dominant hormone and progesterone is deficient, estrogen can potentially become problematic to the body. Dr. John Lee, the physician and author who became popular with his book *What Your Doctor May Not Tell You About Menopause,* was the most outspoken advocate of using natural progesterone to treat menopausal women in order to correct what he called "estrogen dominance."[10]

The goal of natural progesterone creams, in particular, is to support the waning daily production of progesterone in the body and bring back normal premenopausal levels of the hormone. Higher doses of oral progesterone act to increase levels of progesterone in the body more drastically to actually help improve symptoms such as heavy or irregular bleeding, insomnia, and sometimes mood swings.

In treating menopause, progesterone can be used to relieve selected symptoms and to balance the effects of estrogen supplements on the uterus. It has a critical role in preventing endometrial hyperplasia and uterine cancer. Progesterone is often touted in the natural products marketplace as effective for the prevention and treatment of osteoporosis, but actual clinical trials show that neither oral natural progesterone nor progesterone patches or creams can slow, prevent, or reverse bone loss.

I can't stress enough that if you are peri- or postmenopausal and are taking any form of estrogen, you *must* also be taking a proven form and dosage of progesterone (or progestin) to protect your uterus from hyperplasia and cancer. The exception is women who have had a hysterectomy; they do not need to take progesterone or progestins. However, there are times when adding natural progesterone rather than increasing the dose of the estrogen, even in women without a uterus, may alleviate some menopausal symptoms. Some women's insomnia, fatigue, mood swings, and other menopausal symptoms may be more responsive to the progesterone than the estrogen.

It is important to note that all progestins can have undesired side effects.[11] Premenstrual symptoms such as increased breast tenderness, edema, irritability, and abdominal cramps are fairly frequent, causing as much as 40 percent of women to take their prescriptions improperly. More serious side effects are rare and include high blood pressure, blood clotting, and altered carbohydrate lipid metabolism.[12] If you try the synthetic progestins and find you cannot tolerate them, then natural progesterone is an excellent option. In fact, natural progesterone is a *preferred* option. It not only minimizes these symptoms but also may have a positive effect on cholesterol profiles and help to keep the coronary arteries in the heart dilated.

If you are taking estrogen and are one of the few women who cannot tolerate either the synthetic or natural progesterone, you must be monitored by a primary-care practitioner to avoid certain cancers such as uterine cancer.

Progesterone is available with a prescription, in the form of an oral capsule, sublingual drops or pellets, lozenges, transvaginal and rectal suppositories, and injectables. It is also available over the counter, in a low dose, as a cream.

PROGESTERONE CREAMS

The most popular form of progesterone is the topical cream. The goal of natural progesterone cream is to support the waning daily production of progesterone in the body and keep progesterone at normal levels. The goal is *not* to supply pharmacological levels (higher doses) of oral progesterone. Unfortunately, there is currently considerable confusion and misinformation about progesterone creams. There are two basic categories of creams:

- Those that contain wild yam and no progesterone
- Those that contain diosgenin extract (a phytoestrogen compound) from wild yam that is converted into natural progesterone in a laboratory

There are more than six hundred species of wild yam in the world. The greatest concentration of diosgenin seems to be in Mexican wild yam (*Dioscorea barbasco*). However, because there is no regulation of over-the-counter creams, manufacturer labels are not required to state which species of wild yam has been used or whether the diosgenin has been converted to progesterone. The problem is that the creams that only contain wild yam are not effective as a progesterone agent, because the body cannot convert the diosgenin to progesterone by itself.

The confusion is further exacerbated by the varied strengths of the creams. Wild yam extracts with no progesterone come in formulations of 3, 7, or 10 percent extract of wild yam. The wild yam creams with natural progesterone added also come in a wide range of dosages. Some of these products will have less than 2 mg of progesterone per ounce of cream, some may have between 2 and 15 mg per ounce, and some may have as much as 400 mg per ounce. It is important to know exactly what you are getting because the strength of the progesterone will dictate how it is used and what symptoms it should be used for.

As a practitioner, I largely use the creams that have more than 400 mg per ounce because they yield the best results for most women suffering from PMS, menopausal symptoms, and irregular bleeding. In general, however, natural progesterone cream tends to be effective for more mild symptoms of menopause.

Overall, women tolerate natural progesterone cream extremely well, and many find it effective for alleviating some menopausal symptoms. Very few women experience side effects (reported as less than 4 percent by the manufacturing companies), but these may include breast tenderness, drowsiness, depressive moods, headaches, and irritability. And in my experience as a clinician, I have found very few side effects.

Natural progesterone cream is typically used for menopausal symptoms such as hot flashes, mood swings, sleep disruption, and irregular and/or heavy bleeding. I do not recommend use of the cream to prevent heart disease, osteoporosis, breast cancer, endometrial hyperplasia, or uterine cancer. There is continuing research on the benefits of progesterone cream, but to date there is no evidence that it protects women from any of these conditions.

Dose Recommendations

Natural progesterone creams (400 mg progesterone per ounce) for perimenopausal women:
Days 1–7: Do not use progesterone cream during menses.
Days 8–21: Apply ¼ teaspoon of cream to the palms, inner upper arms, or inner thighs twice a day.
Days 22–28: Apply ¼ to ½ teaspoon of cream to any of the same areas twice a day.

Natural progesterone creams (400 mg progesterone per ounce) for menopausal or postmenopausal women:
Apply ¼ teaspoon of cream to the palms, inner upper arms, or inner thighs twice a day.

ORAL MICRONIZED PROGESTERONE (OMP)

While natural progesterone creams are popular with women in menopause, only the oral (and injectable and vaginal gel available by prescription only) forms are available in high enough concentrations to protect against endometrial hyperplasia. Initially, oral progesterone did not absorb into the body very well, which limited its effects. However, today natural progesterone is made through a process called micronization, whereby compounds are pulverized into small particles that are more easily absorbed by the body.

Studies demonstrate that oral micronized progesterone (OMP) is effective in preventing endometrial hyperplasia associated with estrogen use.[13] It does not undermine estrogen's bone loss benefits (nor does it improve bone density when it is added to estrogen replacement),[14] and it does not appear to increase the risk of heart disease.[15]

OMP is available by prescription from a compounding natural pharmacy in any dose your provider prescribes. It is also available from a conventional pharmacy under the trade name Prometrium. In perimenopausal women who are taking estrogen every day, oral progesterone can be given at a dose of 100 mg per day, every day, or it can be given 200 mg per day, days fifteen to twenty-six of the cycle.

These doses are based on an average dose of estrogen replacement or less. For higher doses of estrogen, the dose of progesterone will need to be increased as well, typically doubled. Progesterone is prescribed on a cyclical basis (as opposed to every day) for women who are still bleeding. This cycling of the progesterone allows them to still have a monthly period, the onset of which occurs within a few days of stopping the progesterone.

Dose Recommendations

1. OMP in a perimenopausal woman who is taking continuous estrogen and/or a monthly menstrual cycle is desired: 100 mg twice daily (or 200 mg once daily) twelve days per month.
2. OMP in a perimenopausal woman who is taking estrogen and/or a monthly menstrual cycle is desired: 1 mg estradiol (or equivalent) + OMP 50 mg twice daily (or 100 mg once daily) three weeks on and one week off (during menses).
3. OMP in a postmenopausal woman who is taking continuous estrogen and a monthly cycle is not desired: 1 mg estradiol (or equivalent) + OMP 50 mg twice daily (or 100 mg once daily) continuously.

In my experience, women have few side effects with OMP in doses of 200 mg or less. Higher doses, 400 mg per day, are sometimes prescribed for the diagnosis of amenorrhea, or lack of menstruation, in women who are not yet truly menopausal, or to manage heavy acute uterine bleeding. However, in high doses it can cause side effects including dizziness, abdominal cramping, headaches, breast pain, nausea, diarrhea, fatigue, irritability, and abdominal bloating.[16]

SUBLINGUAL PROGESTERONE

Sublingual (under-the-tongue) progesterone has basically the same uses for premenstrual and menopausal symptoms as the creams and the oral. However, it is generally stronger than the creams and weaker than the usual oral doses. Typically, the tablets, which have a slightly bitter taste, must remain under the tongue for twenty minutes while they dissolve, before the progesterone is fully absorbed.

One advantage of sublingual tablets—as well as creams and vaginal and rectal suppositories—is that they are not significantly metabolized by the liver, as oral progesterone is. This is thought to minimize side effects. However, there is very little information available as to how sublingual progesterone works and what its possible longer-term side effects may be, so I take care when recommending this form of progesterone. Keep in mind that sublingual progesterone and progesterone creams have not been proven to protect the uterus from the effects of estrogen replacement.

Androgens

Androgens are steroid hormones, like testosterone, that control the development and maintenance of masculine characteristics, and provide the source material for a woman's estrogen. A woman's body produces androgens but to a much lesser degree than a man's body. Prior to menopause, androgens, mostly testosterone, are produced by the ovaries and adrenal glands.

Androgens are important for maintaining bone density and sex drive. Your ovaries still produce testosterone postmenopause, but your androgen production decreases by as much as 50 percent from your premenopausal days. This reduction is partly responsible for some common menopausal symptoms such as hot flashes, night sweats, and insomnia. In my experience, women who don't respond to estrogen replacement at conventional dosages may have more relief from their symptoms when they switch to an estrogen/androgen (usually testosterone) combination. You may take testosterone by itself, but it works best when taken with estrogen. Natural testosterone is available from a compounding pharmacy or in a synthetic form called methyltestosterone.

Estrogen/Testosterone Combinations

Estrogen and testosterone therapy is used to improve symptoms like hot flashes and night sweats as well as to improve vaginal dryness, sexual desire, and sexual satisfaction. My clinical experience treating menopausal women with natural testosterone and natural estrogen is quite extensive. Testosterone with estrogen appears to relieve symptoms such as low sexual desire and low arousal more effectively than estrogen alone.

In a number of studies, sexual desire, satisfaction, and frequency of sexual activity were increased when menopausal women switched from HRT (estrogen-only) to an estrogen/testosterone combination.[17] Overall symptom relief was also greater with estrogen/testosterone therapy than with estrogen-only therapy and included a reduction in the intensity of hot flashes and a lessening of vaginal dryness.[18]

There have been some concerns about estrogen/testosterone therapy reversing the higher HDL cholesterol levels achieved with estrogen alone, but the results of studies have been mixed. Further research is needed before it is possible to determine the actual impact on cardiovascular disease. My recommendation: If you are prescribed an estrogen/testosterone combination drug, it would be prudent to have your health-care provider monitor your blood lipid levels to prevent any adverse effects.

Combination estrogen/testosterone therapy may produce a more significant increase in bone density compared with estrogen therapy alone.

Natural testosterone is available in many dosage forms, including oral capsules, injections, and topical preparations. You can buy oral natural testosterone, by prescription, from a compounding pharmacy. I generally use 1 to 6 mg of oral testosterone. Doses in the range of 4 to 6 mg of natural testosterone are considered average physiological doses for women, which I add to a standard bi-estrogen or tri-estrogen formulation (see page 128 for the doses). The combination pills should be taken 1 capsule twice daily.

Testosterone is also available in a cream that can be applied to the genital area to increase sexual response. The cream is typically applied to the external genital area right before sex. Common prescriptions are genital creams that contain 2 mg of testosterone per 16 g of cream. (A good resource for more information about menopause and sexual desire is a book called *The Hormone of Desire* by S. Rako.[19])

Side effects from the use of natural testosterone in the doses given here are rare (estimated to be less than 1 percent). When side effects do occur at these low doses, they can include facial hair growth, acne, hair thinning, and irritability. Abnormally high doses of testosterone can cause side effects such as significant growth of facial and body hair and deepening of the voice.

DHEA

Dehydroepiandrosterone (DHEA) is a natural hormone and another of the androgens. It is the most abundant circulating steroid in humans. DHEA is called a precursor hormone because other steroid hormones, including estrogen and testosterone, are made from it. It was once believed to be inert in the body, but recently there has been interest in its therapeutic effects. In a woman, 90 percent of DHEA comes from the adrenal glands; the remaining 10 percent is manufactured by the ovaries. DHEA is produced at peak levels around age twenty-five and then declines gradually to only 15 to 20 percent of our maximum by the time we turn seventy.

Many claims have been made about the effects of DHEA on the immune system, and its anti-aging effects are said to include better memory, less fatigue, more energy, relaxation, and increased ability to handle stress. It is also touted as having positive effects on bone density and helping to prevent cancer and cardiovascular disease. However, the exact effect DHEA has on the body's cells is unclear. I have seen DHEA increase energy, improve stress response, improve muscle mass, and occasionally increase libido.

A daily oral intake of 50 mg of DHEA for a postmenopausal woman may restore DHEA levels to those of a young adult. At this dosage, DHEA is converted to other more potent androgens, including testosterone. In pharmacologic doses of 1,600 mg, DHEA is converted to estrone and estradiol. Unfortunately, there are only a handful of randomized placebo-controlled studies examining the effects of giving DHEA to humans. Although animal studies are promising, we still need more research on its particular effects on postmenopausal women.

One of the most significant effects of DHEA may be its ability to create a sense of general well-being. Few adverse effects have been reported with DHEA, although androgenic side effects such as facial hair growth and acne can occur with doses as low as 50 mg. A dose of 25 mg daily is more appropriate in my mind; I typically prescribe 5 to 20 mg per day, depending on the severity of the symptoms.

Conclusion

The symptoms of hormone imbalance are well known to those millions of women who suffer from hot flashes, depression, night sweats, insomnia, mood swings, and loss of libido. In the past, hormone replacement therapy has relied on synthetic hormones or animal-derived hormone products that come only in one-size-fits-all doses. While this therapy has worked for some women, many others have found that it had no effect or, worse, that it caused a host of unpleasant side effects. This should be no surprise, since every woman's hormonal profile and needs are unique.

Natural hormone therapy offers a promising alternative to other conventional HRT. However, there is still much to be learned about natural hormones. Further research is needed to study the effects of natural hormones on menopausal symptoms as well as their possible positive and/or negative effects on a woman's breasts, uterus, and cardiovascular system. Using hormones that are identical to those that occur naturally in our bodies is a logical approach to menopause management for many women and their health-care practitioners.

Unfortunately, the bulk of the research on hormone replacement therapy in menopausal women has been conducted using conjugated equine estrogen. What we know to be the negative effects of HRT are associated with these synthetic regimens. What we do not know is if the data translates to natural hormone therapy as well.

If you are using hormones—whether conjugated equine, synthetic, or natural—you should evaluate your hormone regimen with your health-care provider on a regular basis to establish the lowest dose necessary to achieve the benefits and minimize any risks. You should also regularly (at least once a year) discuss how long you should remain on hormone therapy, considering the possible risks.

A truly holistic approach to menopause incorporates the use of hormone therapy, when indicated, in combination with nutritional and botanical supplements and good lifestyle choices such as exercising and adopting a healthy diet. However, many women I have worked with are able to achieve menopausal symptom relief using the nonhormone therapies discussed throughout this book, without ever needing hormone therapy.

6 Osteoporosis Is Not an Inevitable Part of Aging

Rebecca Seguin, M.S., CSCS,
and Miriam Nelson, Ph.D.

Rebecca Seguin is project manager for the John Hancock Center for Physical Activity and Nutrition at the Gerald J. and Dorothy R. Friedman School of Nutrition and Policy at Tufts University in Boston. She received her bachelor's degree in clinical exercise physiology from Boston University and her master's degree in nutrition communication from the Friedman School, where she is now completing her doctorate. Seguin is lead author of the booklet Growing Stronger: Strength Training for Older Adults, *funded by the Centers for Disease Control and Prevention. She is a personal trainer with certification from the National Strength and Conditioning Association and also develops exercise programs for individuals with multiple sclerosis, arthritis, diabetes, osteoporosis, obesity, cardiovascular disease, and other chronic conditions. In addition, Seguin is a freelance health writer, whose work appears in numerous professional and lay press publications. She collaborates with Dr. Miriam Nelson on a variety of projects and has contributed to several chapters in Dr. Nelson's* Strong Women *series.*

Miriam Nelson is author of the internationally best-selling book Strong Women Stay Young; Strong Women Stay Slim; Strong Women, Strong*

Bones; Strong Women Eat Well; *and* Strong Women and Men Beat Arthritis. *Dr. Nelson is the director of the John Hancock Center for Physical Activity and Nutrition and associate professor of Nutrition at the Gerald J. and Dorothy R. Friedman School of Nutrition Science and Policy at Tufts University in Boston. Dr. Nelson is a fellow of the American College of Sports Medicine, an honor reserved for those who have demonstrated superior leadership and research in the field of exercise. Dr. Nelson's best-selling books, which are published in thirteen languages, have sold more than one million copies worldwide.* Strong Women, Strong Bones *received the esteemed Books for a Better Life Award for best wellness book of 2000 from the Multiple Sclerosis Society. She has been featured on many television and radio shows, including* The Oprah Winfrey Show, Today, Good Morning America, *and* Fresh Air, *and on ABC News, CNN, and the Discovery Channel. For the past twelve years, Dr. Nelson has been a principal investigator of studies on exercise and nutrition for midlife and older adults. In 1994, she was named a Brookdale National Fellow; this prestigious award is given annually to a few young scholars deemed to be future leaders in the study of aging. She was awarded a Bunting Fellowship at the Mary Ingraham Bunting Institute at Radcliffe College for 1997–98. In 1998, Dr. Nelson received the Lifetime Achievement Award from the Massachusetts Governor's Committee on Physical Fitness and Sports.*

What's the first thing that comes to mind when you think of healthy, strong bones? If you were born during the twentieth century, *milk* would probably come to mind. That's because most of us grew up hearing some version of the warning, "If you want to be big and strong, drink your milk!" What our parents were saying is that calcium is important to growing bones and that milk is the best source of calcium. Today we know that there is a wide range of sources of calcium that are as good as or better than milk—yogurt, cheese, tofu, and vegetables such as collard greens and spinach, to name a few (for a more complete list of calcium-rich foods, see the table on pages 155–157).

The strength of your bones depends on their mass and density, and bone density depends in part on the amount of calcium and other minerals bones contain. Our ability to build and maintain healthy bones is complex, and although a good diet is clearly an important factor, there are other elements. Strong bones rely upon sufficient lifelong physical activity; consumption of adequate amounts of minerals such as calcium and magnesium, and vitamins such as C, D, and K; and a number of other lifestyle factors.

Although more than 90 percent of bone is built during childhood and adolescence, the body builds and stores bone until about the age of thirty. By the age of twenty, however, the average woman has acquired 98 percent of her skeletal mass. Then, as part of the natural aging process (in both men and women), bones begin to break down faster than new bones can be formed—for women this is especially true. Between the ages of about forty and fifty, most women experience a decline in bone mass, which may leave them at risk for osteoporosis (literally, "porous bones"), a chronic and progressive bone disease associated with reduced bone density and increased susceptibility to fractures.

It is no coincidence that this is the time when most women's ovaries stop producing estrogen (the hormone that protects against bone loss), and women enter the first stage of menopause. The hormonal changes that women experience, combined in many cases with a decrease in physical activity both before and during menopause, make maintaining strong bones through a healthy lifestyle essential. Other risk factors for osteoporosis include gender, age, race, family history, frame size, and tobacco use and other aspects of lifestyle (for a detailed list, see the table on page 144). Today, ten million Americans have osteoporosis—80 percent are women. And one in two women over age fifty will have an osteoporosis-related fracture in her lifetime, according to the National Osteoporosis Foundation.

But there is good news. Osteoporosis—with its related symptoms, such as loss of height, hunched posture, and brittle bones—was once thought to be a normal part of the aging process but is now considered to be preventable. Scientific research has shown that, in most cases, adopting healthy habits—even later in life—such as exercising and eating healthy foods can preserve bone during the midlife years and help avert the development of osteoporosis later in life. Moreover, adopting healthy lifestyle strategies to combat osteoporosis are effective whether or not you decide to use hormone replacement therapy (HRT); this is good news, given the potential risks of HRT. (For more on hormone replacement therapy, see chapter 2. See chapter 5 for a discussion of natural hormone therapy.)

In this chapter you will learn exercise and nutrition information that is essential for healthy muscles and bones. We provide a detailed exercise program that is designed to be safe and effective combined with simple nutrition strategies for maintaining and improving bone health during menopause and beyond.

Bone Basics

Bone is an active, living tissue similar to the lungs, liver, and kidneys. It is the framework that supports our muscles and protects our internal organs. Two types of tissue make up bone—cortical bone, which comprises about 80 percent of bone mass, and trabecular bone, which makes up the other 20 percent. Cortical bone is the outer, dense layer; trabecular bone is the inner layer and is light, porous, and spongy, which makes it considerably more vulnerable to fractures. Depending on the specific bone, the proportion of cortical to trabecular bone varies. The hip, spine, and wrist, for instance, are primarily trabecular bone—that is why these bones are the most common sites of osteoporotic fracture.

As we get older, we are continually growing, adapting, and changing—the same goes for our bones. The process by which bones grow and change is part bone creation (formation), part bone removal (resorption)—collectively called bone remodeling. During bone formation, cells known as osteoblasts produce a protein matrix that causes the remineralization and creation of new bone. During bone resorption, cells called osteoclasts produce enzymes that absorb and remove bone. The remodeling cycle lasts between three and six months, which is approximately how long it takes for a broken bone to heal.

The osteoblasts and osteoclasts work simultaneously and continuously to create the skeleton that supports our muscles and protects our heart and internal organs. Throughout childhood, adolescence, and our early adult years, more bone formation than resorption is occurring, and with adequate nutrition and physical activity our bones grow longer and become increasingly dense. During our twenties and thirties, the activity of osteoblasts and osteoclasts equalizes and bone density remains relatively constant.

By the time we reach our forties and fifties, unfavorable shifts begin to take place in which there is more bone absorption and removal than bone creation. This change causes the density of our bones to slowly deteriorate. For women, these shifts are due, in large part, to the decreased levels of estrogen associated with menopause. Estrogen keeps osteoclast activity in check; when estrogen levels decrease, less bone-building activity takes place.

Estrogen also has an important role in calcium absorption and vitamin D metabolism—both critical to strong bones. Bone-building cells have more available calcium before menopause because estrogen helps the intestines absorb calcium from food and also promotes conservation of calcium by the kidneys, so less is excreted. In addition, estrogen stimulates activity of vitamin D.

Keeping Your Bones Strong for Life

When bone density is significantly reduced, osteoporosis is the result. Osteoporosis is characterized by increased bone fragility and susceptibility to fractures that can result from a slip and fall or from an activity as simple as lifting a heavy bag of groceries. The fear of falling can be mentally debilitating and restrict basic daily activities for those affected by the disease.

While several medications are effective at improving bone density, prevention is truly the best treatment (for more on specific medications, see the table on pages 149–151). Identifying and understanding your own personal risk factors for osteoporosis is essential to prevention, and

Risk Factors for Osteoporosis		
You Can Control	You Can't Control	Medications*
Body weight	Age	Glucosteroids
Diet	Ethnicity	Anticonvulsants
Eating disorder(s)	Family history of	Heparin
Excessive alcohol	osteoporosis	Lithium
or caffeine intake	Being in or past menopause	
Physical activity	Sex (female)	
Smoking	Being small-boned/thin	
	Specific medical	
	conditions*	
	• Hyperthyroidism	
	• Cushing's syndrome	
	• Type I diabetes	
	• Liver disease	

*These are partial lists of medical conditions and medications that may influence risk for osteoporosis. If you have a chronic condition or take medication on a regular basis, talk to your doctor about your bone health regularly.

you have the power to control many of them, such as smoking, poor diet, and inadequate physical activity—all of which can potentially increase your risk for osteoporosis. Other risk factors you have no control over, such as ethnicity, sex, family history, menopausal status, and chronic diseases like hyperthyroidism. However, there are things you can do to minimize the effects of these factors as well. We will be discussing strategies throughout this chapter. See the table above for a list of risk factors and how each is related to osteoporosis.

Bone Density Testing

You may be wondering if you are a candidate for a bone density test and, if so, when you should have your first one. Bone density accounts for about 80 percent of the strength of your bones, and bone density is the best single predictor of future fractures. The best bone density tests predict fractures more successfully than cholesterol levels predict heart attacks or blood pressure predicts stroke. Yet these tests are underutilized, and insurance doesn't always cover them. As a result, less than 10 percent of people with significant bone loss are aware of their problem. As important as these tests are, not everyone needs to be tested right now. Should you have a bone density test? The answer is yes if:

- You have symptoms that suggest osteoporosis, such as bone fractures or loss of height.
- You're beginning hormone replacement therapy or other treatment for your bones or you're planning to stop HRT.
- You have significant risk factors other than being a woman.
- You're in perimenopause or menopause.

Unfortunately, there are usually no symptoms of bone loss. You may not even know you have osteoporosis until your bones become so brittle that they simple break. Once bones have been weakened by osteoporosis, however, you may have signs and symptoms that include back pain, loss of height, and fractures of the vertebrae, wrists, or hips. By the time you reach age fifty, your bone health should be assessed by your doctor. Your doctor will ask you a variety of questions about your lifestyle and medical and family history to determine whether you have osteoporosis or are at risk for the disease. Your doctor will want to know whether anyone in your family suffers from osteoporosis or has had fractured bones. If your risk is high and/or you have already had a fracture—especially after minimal trauma—your physician may recommend a bone density test.

The most common method for assessing bone mineral density (BMD) is a painless, noninvasive imaging technique called dual-energy X-ray absorptiometry (DXA), because it is precise and the dose of radiation is minimal—about one-tenth of a typical X-ray. Also, with DXA it is possible to test multiple sites such as the hip, spine, and wrist or the entire body at once. Other tests that are available for assessing bone density include single-energy X-ray absorptiometry (SXA); dual- and single-photon absorptiometry (DPA, SPA); computerized axial tomography (CT or CAT scan); ultrasound; radiographic absorptiometry (RA); and peripheral dual-energy X-ray absorptiometry (PDXA). These tests can assess bone density at one or more of the following sites: finger, hand, heel, hip, patella, spine, tibia, total body, and wrist.

A bone density test can cost as much as $300. Your health insurance plan may cover some or all of the cost, depending upon the extent of your coverage, your age, and/or the presence of certain risk factors such as family history of osteoporosis, smoking, small-boned and thin body, early menopause, or history of chronic use of steroids. How often bones need to be tested also varies depending on the person.

BMD, measured as grams per square centimeter (g/cm^2), is described by a T-score or a Z-score (see tables on pages 147 and 148). The T-score compares your bone density with that of a healthy young woman; the Z-score compares your bone density with that of other women your own age. Clinically, a diagnosis of osteoporosis is made if your BMD T-score is 2.5 standard deviations lower than the average bone density of a healthy young adult (also defined as bone loss of 25 percent or more). Between 1 and 2.5 standard deviations below normal is clinically defined as osteopenia, a reduction in bone volume to below normal levels but not yet to the point of osteoporosis (with osteopenia, risk for fracture is doubled; with osteoporosis, risk is tripled). If your T-score is higher than –1, your bone density is within 1 standard deviation of that of average, healthy young women and is considered adequate.

Whether you are perimenopausal, going through menopause, or have already begun postmenopause, there are several things you can do to help maintain the bone you currently have and, in many cases, build new bone. Later in this chapter, we discuss exercise and nutritional strategies

		Your Bone Density Compared with That of Younger Women		
T-Score	Statistically Speaking	What It Means to You	Diagnosis
Higher than –1	Your bone mass is within 1 standard deviation (or better) of the average for healthy young adult women.	Your bone mass and your risk of fractures are average or better; 85% of healthy young women are in this range.	Adequate bone density
Between –1 and –2.5	Your bone mass is between 1 and 2.5 standard deviations lower than the average for healthy young adult women.	Your bone mass is lower than normal, and your fracture risk is approximately twice as high as average. The lowest 1–14% of healthy young adult women have bone density in this range.	Osteopenia
Less than –2.5	Your bone mass is lower than the average for healthy young adult women by more than 2.5 standard deviations.	Your bone density is very low—lower than that of 99% of healthy young adult women. Your risk of fractures is about three times higher than average.	Osteoporosis

to bolster bone health, including specific recommendations for those of you who may already have low BMD. If your BMD testing reveals osteopenia or osteoporosis, there are also medication options you may want to consider. The information we provide here (see the table on pages 149–151) comes from the most up-to-date recommendations (at the time of this publishing) from the National Osteoporosis Foundation (www.nof.org). Keep in mind, though, that new medications for prevention and treatment frequently become available. It is crucial that you continue to discuss the available options with your health-care provider, on the basis of your own individual needs.

Your Bone Density Compared with That of Women Your Own Age		
Z-Score	Statistically Speaking	What It Means to You
Higher than –1	Your bone mass is within 1 standard deviation of the average for women your age, or better.	Your bone mass is within or above the normal range for women your age.
Between –1 and –2.5	Your bone mass is between 1 and 2.5 standard deviations lower than the average for women your age.	Your bone mass is lower than average for your age. Compared with your peers, you're in the lowest 1–14%.
Less than –2.5	Your bone mass is lower by more than 2.5 standard deviations than the average for women your age.	Your bone density is much lower than average—lower than that of 99% of women your age.

Good Nutrition for Healthy Bones

Whether you eat meat and consume dairy products on a regular basis or you are a vegetarian, achieving a bone-healthy diet is easier than you may think. If you are a vegan, you will need to pay special attention to getting adequate calcium through fortified options such as soy, juices, and others foods. If necessary, you can take a supplement to fill in the gap. The following section discusses important minerals and vitamins.

CALCIUM

Calcium makes up a considerable portion of our bone mass and is fundamental for strong bones. It is also essential for bodily functions such as nerve transmission, muscle contraction, and blood pressure regulation. To maintain these activities and to ensure proper function of the bone remodeling process, you must regularly consume an adequate amount of calcium, by

Medication Options for Low Bone Density and Indications for Their Use

Category	Name	Comments
Bisphosphonate	Alendronate sodium (brand name Fosamax)	*Prevention:* 5 mg/day or 35 mg once per week *Treatment:* 10 mg/day or 70 mg once per week *Action:* reduces bone loss; increases BMD; reduces risk of fracture *Side effects:* uncommon, but may include abdominal or musculoskeletal pain, nausea, heartburn, irritation of the esophagus *Special notes:* • Must be taken on an empty stomach first thing in the morning with 8 ounces of water; must remain upright and abstain from other food and drink for at least 30 minutes afterward • Also approved for men with osteoporosis
Bisphosphonate	Risedronate sodium (brand name Actonel)	*Prevention:* 5 mg/day or 35 mg once per week *Treatment:* 10 mg/day or 70 mg once per week *Action:* reduces bone loss; increases BMD; reduces risk of fracture *Side effects:* uncommon, but may include abdominal or musculoskeletal pain, nausea, heartburn, irritation of the esophagus *Special notes:* • Must be taken on an empty stomach first thing in the morning with 8 ounces of water; must remain upright and abstain from other food and drink for at least 30 minutes afterward • Also approved for men with osteoporosis *(continued)*

Category	Name	Comments
Hormone	Calcitonin (brand name Miacalcin)	*Prevention and treatment:* 200 units nasal spray once per day *Action:* increases bone mass *Side effects:* from injection—side effects may include flushing of the face and hands, urinary frequency, nausea, and a skin rash; from nasal spray (uncommon)—nasal irritation, backache, bloody nose, and headaches *Special notes:* • For women more than 5 years beyond menopause • Must be taken via a daily injection or nasal spray
SERM (selective estrogen receptor modulators)	Raloxifene (brand name Evista)	*Prevention and treatment:* 60 mg a day (pill form, with or without meals), for postmenopausal osteoporosis *Action:* increases bone mass; reduces risk of spine fractures *Side effects:* hot flashes, venous thrombotic events
Parathyroid Hormone	Teriparatide (brand name Fortéo)	*Prevention and treatment:* self-administered as a daily injection; for postmenopausal women and men at high risk for a fracture *Action:* stimulates new bone formation; increases bone mineral density in the spine, hip, foot, ribs, and wrist in postmenopausal women; in men, fracture reduction noted in the spine *Side effects:* nausea, leg cramps, dizziness
Hormone Replacement Therapy	Estrogen Replacement Therapy (ERT)/ Hormone Replacement Therapy (HRT) (many brand names)	*Prevention:* low dose: 0.3mg/day; standard dose: 0.625mg/day

Category	Name	Comments
Hormone Replacement Therapy	Estrogen Replacement Therapy (ERT)/ Hormone Replacement Therapy (HRT) (many brand names)	*Action:* ERT has been shown to reduce bone loss, increase bone density in both the spine and hip, and reduce the risk of hip and spinal fractures in postmenopausal women. ERT is administered most commonly in the form of a pill or skin patch that delivers a low dose of approximately 0.3 mg daily or a standard dose of approximately 0.625 mg daily.
		Important Note: Studies have shown that estrogen, when taken alone, can increase risk for endometrial cancer, so it is prescribed with progesterone to eliminate that risk. In addition, new research has confirmed that HRT increases risk for breast cancer, stroke, heart attack, and blood clots (see chapter 2). The FDA currently advises that when prescribing solely for the prevention of postmenopausal osteoporosis, therapy should only be considered for women at a significant risk of osteoporosis, and non-estrogen medications should be carefully considered.
		Other side effects: vaginal bleeding, breast tenderness, mood disturbances, and gallbladder disease

way of a proper diet or through supplementation. When you don't, your body saps the skeleton of its calcium to maintain these vital functions. If dietary intake is inadequate for a substantial length of time, your bones suffer.

For women aged nineteen to fifty years, the current dietary reference intake (or DRI, the term that has replaced the previously used "recommended daily allowance," or RDA) is 1,000 milligrams (mg)/day; for women aged fifty-one years and older, the DRI is 1,200 mg/day (see the table on page 155). Surveys show that many Americans are not getting enough calcium—many women consume less than half the daily recommended amount. Later in this chapter, we suggest food options and strategies for consuming a diet that is rich in calcium as well as other bone-essential nutrients (see the tables on pages 155–163).

If you are unable to get enough calcium in your diet (this may be especially true for those who are lactose intolerant), ask your doctor to recommend a calcium supplement. Calcium is available in two main types: calcium carbonate and calcium citrate. Calcium carbonate tends to be slightly less expensive and the pills are a bit smaller. The downside is that it must be taken with food and that it causes gas and/or constipation in some people. Calcium citrate is a little more expensive than calcium carbonate, but it is better absorbed; does not typically cause bloating, gas, or constipation; and can be taken on a full or empty stomach.

A person's ability to absorb calcium effectively can be affected by dietary factors such as too much protein, caffeine, or sodium, which can increase the amount of calcium excreted in urination. Adding fiber to foods or drinking fiber supplement drinks can also decrease calcium absorption because foods travel through the digestive system too quickly for the calcium to be absorbed.

VITAMIN D

Vitamin D is an equally essential nutrient for strong bones. Without it we cannot absorb the calcium we consume, and the process by which calcium is made into bone is compromised. We get some vitamin D from our diet (or from supplements), and vitamin D is also manufactured in the skin through direct exposure to the sun. Typically, ten to fifteen minutes of exposure to sunlight two to three times a week is sufficient to guarantee enough vitamin D.

However, starting around age fifty, our bodies do not absorb vitamin D or make it from the sun as easily as they once did. Therefore, it is important to make sure you get enough vitamin D from food or supplements (see the table on page 162).

Ample amounts of vitamin D do not naturally occur in many foods. The major food sources of vitamin D are fortified dairy products; egg yolks; cold saltwater fish and seafood such as Atlantic mackerel, halibut, herring, oysters, salmon, shrimp, and tuna. In cold climates where the sun's rays are weaker several months of the year, the body cannot make vitamin D on its own.

To recap: The limited availability of vitamin D in foods, seasonal factors, age-related reductions in absorption, and the fact that vitamin D is absolutely necessary for bone health make this a supplement you should consider starting at the age of forty (see the table on page 155). For women aged fifty-one to seventy, the DRI is 400 International Units (IU) or 10 micrograms (mcg)/day; aged seventy-one and older, the DRI is 600 IU or 15 mcg/day. You should not be getting more than 50 mcg (or 2,000 IU) of vitamin D per day—and 800 IUs is plenty. Depending on your dietary intake of calcium, you might consider a calcium plus vitamin D supplement or a vitamin D supplement on its own. Just keep in mind that too much of something can be as harmful as not enough. Excess vitamin D can be toxic, so take a look at your diet first and see whether you are getting enough there before taking supplements.

Important findings published in the September 2000 *American Journal of Clinical Nutrition* by Dr. Bess Dawson-Hughes and colleagues at Tufts University demonstrate that you must continue to take your supplements to achieve long-term benefit for bones. Men and women (sixty-eight years and older) who participated in a three-year randomized, controlled trial of calcium and vitamin D supplementation at our research center experienced significant increases in bone mineral density over the three years—with a significant reduction in fractures. Researchers then followed these volunteers for another two years while they did not take the supplements. They found that the majority of bone benefits were completely lost during the two years without supplementation.[1]

MAGNESIUM AND POTASSIUM

These two nutrients have an important role in numerous bodily functions as well as bone health. Fortunately, you can easily consume adequate amounts through your diet (see the tables on pages 157–159). Fruit and vegetables are excellent sources of both; whole grains are a good source of magnesium; and milk and yogurt supply a fair amount of potassium. There are no conclusive studies to support taking supplements of either of these nutrients for bone or general health as long you are eating a healthy diet. The DRI for magnesium is 350 mg/day; there is no DRI for potassium, just a Daily Value (DV)—not a value for recommended intake but a general idea of how much of a vitamin or mineral a serving of a given food contributes to the total daily diet—which is 3,500 mg/day (see the table on page 155).

VITAMINS C AND K

Vitamins C and K play a critical role in collagen production, which is the first stage in building new bone. The DRI for vitamin C is 60 mg/day, and the DRI for vitamin K is 70 mcg/day (see the table on page 155)—although preliminary research shows that consuming higher quantities of both may be beneficial to bone. You can consume plenty of vitamin C through fruit (especially citrus fruit) and vegetables. Foods such as broccoli, Brussels sprouts, spinach, and collard greens are excellent sources of vitamin K (see the tables on pages 160–161).

If you are concerned about one or more nutrients or you are interested in easy ways to boost the nutrient content of your diet, look at the ten bone-healthy nutrition tips in the table on page 163.

Dietary Reference Intake (DRI) of Vitamins and Nutrients Related to Bone Health

Nutrient	Recommended Daily Intake
Calcium	
19–50 years of age	1,000 mg/day
51 years and older	1,200 mg/day
Vitamin D	
Birth to age 50	200 IU or 5 mcg/day*
51–70 years of age	400 IU or 10 mcg/day
71 years and older	600 IU or 15 mcg/day
Magnesium	350 mg/day
Potassium	3,500 mg/day (DV)
Vitamin C	60 mg/day
Vitamin K	70 mcg/day

*40 IU = 1 mcg

Nutrient-Rich Foods—Based on the United States Department of Agriculture (USDA) National Nutrient Database

Foods Rich in Calcium

Food	Serving Size	Value (mg)
DAIRY PRODUCTS AND SOY MILK		
Ricotta cheese, whole milk	1 cup	500
Yogurt, plain, low-fat	8 ounces	415
Milk (whole, low-fat, or skim)	1 cup	270–300

(continued)

Food	Serving Size	Value (mg)
Hard cheese high in calcium: Swiss, provolone, cheddar, Monterey Jack, Parmesan, Romano, part-skim mozzarella	1 ounce	200–300
Hard and soft cheeses with medium calcium levels: American, Gouda, Colby, whole-milk mozzarella, feta, fontina, blue, Camembert	1 ounce	100–200
Soft cheeses low in calcium: Brie, Neufchâtel, cream cheese	1 ounce	20–50
Cottage cheese (whole-milk, low-fat)	1 cup	130–160
Ice cream and frozen yogurt	½ cup	70–120
Milk-based puddings and custards	½ cup	150
Soy milk, calcium fortified	1 cup	200–300
Soy milk, not calcium fortified	1 cup	10
SOY AND OTHER BEANS		
Tofu made with calcium sulfate	1 cup	500
Tofu made without calcium sulfate	1 cup	250
Soybeans, dry roasted, soy nuts	1 cup	450
Soybeans, green, cooked	1 cup	260
Texturized vegetable protein	1 cup	170
Tempeh	1 cup	150
Miso paste	½ cup	90
Kidney beans, chickpeas, navy beans, pinto beans, green beans	1 cup	50–120

Food	Serving Size	Value (mg)
VEGETABLES		
Collards, cooked	1 cup	350
Spinach	1 cup	300
Turnip greens	1 cup	250
Kale, cooked	1 cup	180
Okra, cooked	1 cup	175
Cabbage, cooked	1 cup	160
Broccoli	1 cup	60
FISH		
Sardines, canned, with bones	3 ounces	325
Salmon, canned, with bones	3 ounces	180
Halibut	½ fillet	95
Trout	3 ounces	75
Haddock	1 fillet	65

Foods Rich in Magnesium

Food	Serving Size	Value (mg)
Trail mix (chocolate chips, salted nuts, seeds)	1 cup	235
Spinach, cooked	1 cup	157
Pumpkin seeds	1 ounce	151
Black beans, cooked	1 cup	120
Artichoke, cooked	1 cup	100
Halibut, cooked	3 ounces	91
Oat bran muffin	1 muffin	89
Great northern beans, cooked	1 cup	89
Chickpeas, cooked	1 cup	79

Food	Serving Size	Value (mg)
Grapefruit juice	6 fluid ounces	79
Nuts (cashews, almonds)	1 ounce	77
Lentils, cooked	1 cup	71
Split peas, cooked	1 cup	71
Potato, baked with skin	1 potato	57
Tuna or Yellowfish, cooked	3 ounces	54
Peanuts, all types, dry roasted	1 ounce	50
Soy milk	1 cup	47
Raisins, seedless	1 cup	46
Yogurt, plain, skim milk	1 cup	43
Banana	1 cup	41
Tomato products, canned	1 cup	39
Peanuts, roasted	½ cup	131
Tofu, raw, regular	½ cup	127
Broccoli stalks, cooked	2 large	120
Spinach, cooked	½ cup	79
Swiss chard, cooked	½ cup	76
Soybeans, cooked	½ cup	74
Sweet potato, cooked	½ cup	61
Black beans, cooked	½ cup	60
White beans, cooked	½ cup	57
Baked beans	½ cup	55
Peanut butter	2 tablespoons	51
Artichoke, cooked	1 medium	47
Pinto beans, cooked	½ cup	47
Acorn squash, baked	½ cup	43
Chickpeas, cooked	½ cup	39
Yogurt, low-fat	1 cup	37

Foods Rich in Potassium

Food	Serving Size	Value (mg)
Orange juice, frozen concentrate	6 fluid ounces	1,435
Beans, white, canned	1 cup	1,189
Tomato products, canned, puréed	1 cup	1,098
Raisins, seedless	1 cup	1,086
Potato, baked with skin	1 potato	1,080
Grapefruit juice, frozen concentrate	6 fluid ounces	1,002
Squash, winter, baked	1 cup	896
Spinach, cooked	1 cup	839
Papaya	1 papaya	781
Baked beans	1 cup	752
Lentils, cooked	1 cup	730
Split peas, cooked	1 cup	710
Sweet potato, cooked	1 potato	694
Artichoke, cooked	1 cup	595
Banana	1 cup	557
Yogurt, plain, low-fat	1 cup	531
Beets, cooked	1 cup	519
Halibut, cooked	3 ounces	490
Tuna or Yellowfish, cooked	3 ounces	484
Broccoli, cooked	1 cup	457
Apricots, dried	10 halves	408
Sauerkraut, canned	1 cup	401
Milk, whole	1 cup	370

Foods Rich in Vitamin C

FOOD	SERVING SIZE	VALUE (MG)
Orange juice, frozen concentrate	6 fluid ounces	294
Peppers, sweet, red	1 cup	283
Grapefruit juice, frozen concentrate	6 fluid ounces	248
Peaches, frozen, sliced	1 cup	236
Papaya, raw	1 papaya	188
Strawberries, raw	1 cup	98
Brussels sprouts, cooked	1 cup	97
Cranberry juice	8 fluid ounces	90
Broccoli, raw	1 cup	78
Kiwi fruit	1 medium	70
Orange	1 orange	70
Soup, tomato	1 cup	68
Cantaloupe	1 cup	59
Mango	1 mango	57
Cauliflower, cooked	1 cup	56
Pineapple	1 cup	56
Kale, cooked	1 cup	53
Cabbage, cooked	1 cup	44
Asparagus, cooked	1 cup	44
Chestnuts, roasted	1 cup	37
Beet, turnip, mustard greens	1 cup	35
Raspberries, raw	1 cup	32
Lemons, raw, without peel	1 cup	31
Honeydew melon	⅛ melon	29
Sweet potato, cooked	1 potato	29
Tangerine	1 tangerine	26
Tomato, red, ripe, raw	1 cup	23

Foods Rich in Vitamin K		
FOOD	SERVING SIZE	VALUE (MCG)
Kale or collards, cooked	1 cup	1,060
Spinach, cooked	1 cup	888
Brussels sprouts, cooked	1 cup	300
Broccoli, cooked	1 cup	220
Lettuce, butterhead	1 head	167
Noodles, egg or spinach, cooked	1 cup	162
Asparagus, cooked	1 cup	144
Sauerkraut, canned	1 cup	135
Lettuce, green leaf	1 cup	97
Cabbage, cooked	1 cup	73
Cucumber, raw, with peel	1 large	50
Peas, cooked	1 cup	48
Blueberries, frozen	1 cup	40
Tuna, light, canned in oil	3 ounces	37
Kiwi fruit	1 medium	30
Blackberries, raw	1 cup	29
Artichokes, cooked	1 cup	25

Foods Rich in Vitamin D
(not included in USDA National Nutrient Database)

Food	Serving Size	Value (IU)
NATURAL SOURCES		
Herring	3 ounces	1,383
Herring, pickled	3 ounces	578
Salmon, canned	3 ounces	530
Halibut	3 ounces	510
Cod liver oil	1 teaspoon	450
Catfish	3 ounces	425
Mackerel, Atlantic	3 ounces	306
Oysters	3 ounces	272
Shiitake mushrooms, dried	4 mushrooms	249
Sardines, canned in oil	½ cup	203
Tuna, light meat	3 ounces	200
Shrimp	3 ounces	129
FORTIFIED SOURCES		
Tofu, fortified	3 ounces	120
Cow's milk, all types	1 cup	100
Rice milk, fortified	1 cup	100
Soy milk, fortified	1 cup	100
Orange juice, fortified	1 cup	100

10 Bone-Healthy Nutrition Tips

Tips	Nutrient Boost
1. Prepare soups, casseroles, and other dishes with non-fat or reduced-fat milk.	Boosts calcium and vitamin D
2. Have a strawberry-banana yogurt smoothie as an afternoon snack.	Boosts calcium, vitamin C, and potassium
3. Snack on almonds instead of potato chips or pretzels.	Boosts calcium
4. Substitute whole-wheat bread for white.	Boosts magnesium
5. Try baby spinach as the base of your salad instead of lettuce.	Boosts vitamin K and magnesium
6. Top your baked potato with shredded cheddar cheese and broccoli.	Boosts calcium, magnesium, and vitamin K
7. Enjoy a milkshake (regular or calcium-fortified soy milk, ice cream, and your choice of flavoring) for dessert.	Boosts vitamin D and calcium
8. Top your salad or pasta with chilled saltwater fish or seafood (tuna, salmon, or shrimp).	Boosts vitamin D
9. Add barley and brown rice to soups.	Boosts magnesium
10. Enjoy several servings of seasonal fresh fruits and vegetables every day.	Boosts magnesium, potassium, vitamin C, and vitamin K

An Exercise Program for Healthy Bones

We all know that muscle gets stronger and bigger the more it is used. But did you know that bone becomes stronger and denser the more it is worked? Conversely, if bones are not used, through physical activity, particularly as you get older, they will lose mass and density. When combined with good nutrition, specifically targeted exercises can help combat the effect of reduced estrogen levels and diminished bone formation during menopause. Two types of exercise that are important for building and maintaining bone mass and density are weight-bearing exercises (weightlifting, especially for the arms, legs, and torso) and resistance exercises (walking, cycling, stair climbing, and dancing). In addition, by strengthening your muscles and bones, and improving your balance, exercise can help to prevent falls and fractures. One caveat: If you have or suspect you have osteoporosis, it is important to take extra caution when starting an exercise regimen. Consult your doctor first about your risk of fracture.

In general, most physical activity contributes to better health for your body, mind, and spirit; and, in many cases, better bone density. Some types of activity, such as swimming, have not been shown to bolster bone health but have an important role in the prevention of other chronic diseases like heart disease. Similarly, while leisure activities such as golf have not specifically shown a positive effect on bone density, it is likely that they contribute to maintaining healthy bones, because greater levels of physical activity, in general, mean stronger muscles and better overall fitness. For the optimum effect, try to do a minimum of thirty minutes of vigorous (sweat-producing) exercise at least three days per week and an additional thirty to sixty minutes of general physical activity such as cycling, walking, golf, tennis, yoga, Pilates, or swimming on most days of the week.

The following list features different types of activity. The high-impact exercises that are especially helpful in boosting bone density are marked with asterisks. These activities are recommended only with your doctor's approval if you have osteopenia or osteoporosis.

ACTIVITY LIST

Aerobic Exercises

- Running, jogging*
- Kickboxing*
- High-impact (or step) aerobics*
- Low-impact aerobics
- Brisk walking
- Cycling
- Swimming
- Stair climbing
- Elliptical/cross training

Strength-Training Exercises

- Weightlifting with machines or free weights
- Exercises with rubber tubing
- Push-ups
- Squats

Sport and Leisure Activities

- Basketball*
- Volleyball*
- Gymnastics*
- Jumping rope*
- Skipping*
- Tennis
- Golf
- Gardening

Other

- Vertical jumping*
- Yoga
- Pilates
- Flexibility exercises
- Aqua aerobics

Strength Training
for Healthy Bones and Muscles

Because your muscles, bones, and cardiovascular system respond to the amount of physical stress placed upon them, strength training is a perfect activity for maintaining healthy bones. Specific strength-training exercises can target bones in the body that are especially vulnerable to fracture—namely the hip, spine, and wrist.

There is now an extensive body of research illustrating the importance of strength-training exercises for bone health. For example: Scientists at the Mayo Clinic in Rochester, Minnesota, have published a study showing a reduction in fractures with strength training.[2] What is interesting about the study is that the benefits showed up many years after the main study was concluded.

Over a decade ago, the scientists took a group of fifty women (aged fifty-eight to seventy-five) and randomized them into two different groups. One group performed muscle-strengthening exercises of the back muscles for two years, and the other group served as controls. At the end of two years, the women who had been strength training had stronger back muscles, but there was no difference between groups in bone density. Eight years later, the scientists brought the women back into the laboratory to test them to see if any differences still remained. What they saw was dramatic. The women who had originally been strength training still had stronger back muscles, but this time their bone density was better than the controls. Most important, the women in the control group had experienced almost three times as many vertebral fractures (fractures of the bones in the spine) than the women who were originally in the strength-training group. The controls had had fourteen crush fractures, whereas the strength trainers had had only six crush fractures. This was a highly significant difference between groups.

There are literally hundreds of strengthening exercises and variations that are effective for maintaining healthy bones. However, we chose a few specific exercises with three primary goals in mind. The first was to design a program that could be done easily with minimal equipment and without going to the gym. The second was to ensure that the exercises had been proven safe through extensive testing and experience. (We have used these exercises safely in laboratory and home-based settings.) The third was to make sure the program is one that you can do regularly in the least amount of time possible. As you'll see in the example schedules we provide (see pages 183–184), this program—like most physical activity—does not have to be done all at once to be effective. Rather, we encourage you to fit strength training and other physical activities you enjoy into your day-to-day life.

WHAT YOU NEED TO GET STARTED

Among our considerations in designing this program was the need for minimal equipment. This is helpful in two ways: It keeps your costs low, and it limits the amount of storage space you need.

Mandatory Equipment

1. Two to four sets of dumbbells of varying weights. The weights will depend on your level of experience and strength. If you are just beginning, you may want to start with a set of 2-, 3-, and 5-pound dumbbells. If you have used weights previously, a set of 5-, 8-, and 10-pound weights will offer you more of a challenge.
2. Chair and counter or table. You will need a sturdy chair to do the wide-leg squat exercise. You will also need enough space to use a countertop or sturdy table for the lunge exercise.
3. Carpeted floor and/or exercise mat. For several exercises you will be lying on the floor. If the carpet is thick, you may be able to simply place a towel on the carpet. Another option is to purchase an exercise mat.

Optional Equipment

1. Ankle weights. Ankle weights increase the intensity of certain exercises, such as side-leg raises.
2. Storage container or cart to keep the dumbbells and ankle weights out of the way.

TIMING, BREATHING, AND INTENSITY

As you read through the exercises, you may notice that we remind you often to move slowly and to breathe throughout every exercise. This may seem repetitive at first, but breathing is one of the most important aspects of an exercise routine, and it is not always as easy as you would think to maintain a strong, steady breath. In order to reap maximum benefits from your workouts and ensure that you don't injure yourself, move slowly—a full three-second count as you raise the weights and three seconds as you lower them (or longer if you can). Use the same pace if you are doing exercises without weights such as squats, lunges, and sit-ups.

You may have heard that there are specific breathing techniques for strength training—such as breathing out during the lifting phase and breathing in during the lowering phase. Because some people have a tendency to hold their breath when they lift weights, we emphasize that *when* and *how* you breathe are less important than breathing continually throughout each exercise.

If you were exercising at a gym with a personal trainer, you would have strict guidance on posture, technique, and when to increase the weight (intensity) you are lifting. However, if you choose to undertake a home-based strength-training program like this one, you will essentially be your own personal trainer. We recommend that you start out very slowly and conservatively in the beginning. This will allow you to become accustomed to the exercises and avoid injury. As you feel comfortable with the exercises and your strength increases, you can begin lifting heavier weights.

To determine whether or not you are ready to increase the intensity of your workout, ask yourself the following questions:

1. Am I able to complete two sets of ten repetitions using proper form?

No: Reduce the weight load to an amount that you can lift ten times in good form; then repeat for a second set.

Yes: Please continue to question two.

2. After completing ten repetitions, do I need to rest because the weight is too heavy to complete more repetitions using proper form?

Yes: You are working at the proper intensity and should not increase the weight.

No: Please continue to questions three and four to determine how to safely increase the intensity of your workout.

3. Could I have completed a few more repetitions while staying in proper form and without taking a break?

Yes: If you could only do a *few* more repetitions (not the entire next set of ten without a break), do the first set of repetitions with the current weight and your second set with the next weight up at your next workout. For example, if you're currently using 1-pound dumbbells, use 2- or 3-pound dumbbells for the second set.

4. Could I have done all twenty repetitions at one time, without a break?

Yes: At your next session, use heavier dumbbells for both sets of repetitions.

Strength-Training Exercises for Strong Bones

WIDE-LEG SQUAT

This multipurpose exercise (see figure 3) strengthens the muscles of your hips, thighs, and buttocks while also helping to improve your body awareness and balance.

Instructions

1. Stand with your feet pointing slightly outward and greater than hip-width apart in front of a sturdy chair that is either on a rug or against the wall to prevent sliding. Face away from the chair and cross your arms over your chest.
2. Keep your focus straight ahead with shoulders relaxed and chest high. To a count of 3, slowly bend at the hips and knees to lower your buttocks toward the chair—stopping just before you reach a seated position.
3. Remember to breathe.
4. As you lower to and rise up from the chair, keep your weight focused and push up through the heel of your foot; your knees should not drift forward past your toes, which can put stress on your

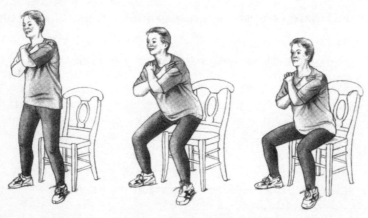

Figure 3: Wide-Leg Squat

knees; if you look down at the floor, you should be able to see the tips of your toes.

5. Pause. Then, to a count of 3, slowly rise to a standing position.
6. Complete 2 sets of 10 repetitions with a break of approximately 1 minute between sets.

If you find this exercise too challenging, put a pillow or two on the chair and lower down into the squat only to the point where your buttocks graze the pillow(s). As you strengthen the muscles of your hips, thighs, and buttocks, you will be able to lower yourself down to just above the seat of the chair.

LUNGE

The lunge (see figure 4) is a versatile, dynamic exercise aimed at strengthening the muscles of your entire leg—calf, thigh, and buttocks. Similar to the wide-leg squat, it is excellent for improving balance and body awareness, which, combined with strengthening of muscles and bones, will help prevent falls and potential fractures.

Instructions

1. Stand with your right hip a few inches from a counter or sturdy table and let your hand gently rest on the counter- or tabletop, keeping your feet together or just slightly separated. Your shoulders should be relaxed and chest high to maintain good posture.
2. Take a large step forward with your right leg. Then, to a count of 3, slowly bend both knees so that your right thigh is about parallel to the ground and your left knee is close to, but not touching, the ground. Your right knee should not move over the toes of your right foot.
3. Remember to breathe.

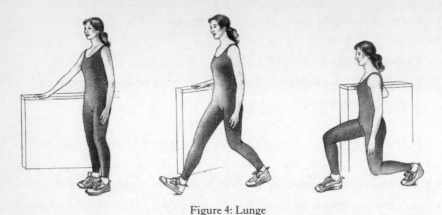

Figure 4: Lunge

4. Keep your upper body erect with your focus straight ahead, shoulders relaxed and chest high. Pause. Then, to a count of 3, slowly push from the right heel to rise back up to the standing position and bring your right foot forward to meet your other foot.
5. Make sure that when you return to the starting position, you push your weight backward rather than upward.
6. Complete 2 sets of 10 repetitions stepping forward with the right leg with a break of approximately 1 minute between sets. Then complete 2 sets of 10 repetitions stepping forward with the left leg.

If you find this exercise too challenging, stick with the wide-leg squat to begin with. When your legs become stronger, add the lunge to your routine.

SIDE-LEG RAISE

The side-leg raise (see figure 5) is a terrific exercise for targeting the muscles and bones of the hip. It can also improve agility by strengthening the muscles of the outer thigh that are essential to good balance, which is important in helping to reduce the risk of falls.

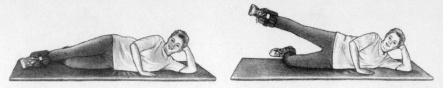

Figure 5: Side-Leg Raise

Instructions

1. If you are using ankle weights, strap one on each leg. (Ankle weights are not mandatory for this exercise; rather, they will add additional challenge when you're ready.)
2. Lie on your side on a carpeted floor or on an exercise mat with your hips stacked. Keep your thighs on top of each other but bend the knee of the bottom leg to stabilize your balance.
3. To a count of 3, keeping the top leg straight, slowly lift your leg away from the floor to a height of 6 to 18 inches. When lifting, let your heel (not your toes) lead your leg.
4. Remember to breathe.
5. Pause. Then, to a count of 3, slowly lower your leg back down to starting position.
6. Complete 2 sets of 10 repetitions lifting the right leg, with a break of approximately 1 minute between sets. Then, complete 2 sets of 10 repetitions lifting the left leg.

ONE-ARM REVERSE FLY

The vast majority of people have suffered from back pain at one time or another. In many cases, weak back muscles are the culprits. This exercise (see figure 6) will strengthen the muscles of your upper back and shoulders, helping you maintain good posture, and reduce stress on the spine.

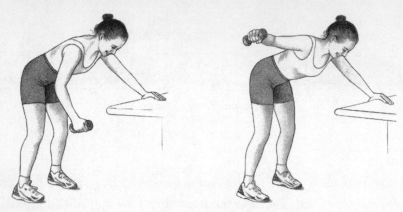

Figure 6: One-Arm Reverse Fly

Instructions

1. Stand with your left hip about 2 feet from a sturdy table or counter with your feet shoulder-width apart. Bend forward at the hip, resting your left hand on the counter or table to stabilize the position.
2. With a dumbbell in your right hand, slowly raise your arm directly out to the side to a count of 3, keeping your elbow relaxed and palm facing down.
3. Remember to breathe.
4. Keep your knees and elbows soft (with a slight bend) throughout this exercise.
5. Make sure that your wrist and forearm as well as your head, neck, and back are in alignment and do not hunch your shoulders.
6. Pause. Then, to a count of 3, lower your arm back to the starting position.
7. Complete 2 sets of 10 repetitions on your right arm, with a break of approximately 1 minute between sets. Then complete 2 sets of 10 repetitions on your left arm.

PUSH-UP

The push-up (see figure 7) is a simple yet practical exercise that many of us remember from our youth. It strengthens the wrists, chest, and shoulders while improving balance and body awareness.

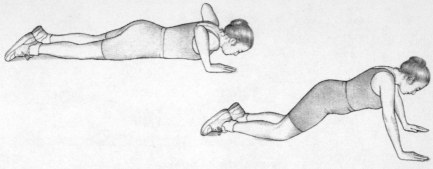

Figure 7: Push-Up

Instructions

1. Lie facedown on a carpeted floor or mat with your hands just to the sides of your shoulders, fingers facing forward and elbows bent and pointing upward.
2. Keeping your knees on the ground and your feet relaxed, slowly push your shoulders, chest, torso, and thighs away from the ground (keeping them all in alignment) to a count of 3.
3. Remember to breathe.
4. Keep your abdominal muscles contracted and make sure your thighs, buttocks, back, head, and neck stay in alignment during this exercise.
5. Place a folded towel under your knees for added cushion if needed.
6. Pause. Then, to a count of 3, slowly lower your body back down until you are hovering just above the starting position.
7. Complete 2 sets of 10 repetitions, with a break of approximately 1 minute between sets.
8. When you're ready for an added challenge, advance this move to the classic push-up—knees off the floor, legs in full alignment, and weight in your hands and toes.

BACK EXTENSION

This simple back extension exercise (see figure 8) will strengthen the small but important erector spinae muscle group that runs along your spine. It

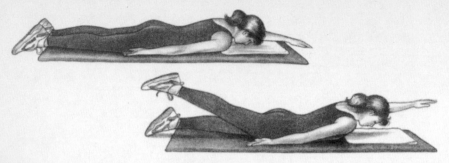

Figure 8: Back Extension

will help avert back pain and enhance posture while targeting the bones of your spine, which are particularly vulnerable to osteoporosis as we age.

Instructions

1. Lie facedown on a carpeted floor or mat with your left arm extended straight above your head and parallel to the floor and your right arm at your side.
2. Keep your gaze at the ground and your head and neck in alignment and slowly lift your left arm and right leg off the ground to a count of 3.
3. Remember to breathe.
4. To ensure that your head and neck stay in alignment during this exercise, keep the lifting arm over your ear.
5. Place a pillow under your knees for added cushion if needed.
6. Pause. Then, to a count of 3, slowly lower your arm and leg back to the ground.
7. Complete 2 sets of 10 repetitions lifting the left arm and right leg, with a break of approximately 1 minute between sets. Then, do 2 sets of 10 repetitions lifting the right arm and left leg with a 1-minute break between sets.

ABDOMINAL CURL

Around the time of menopause, it's not uncommon for women to begin noticing that their tummy isn't as flat as it once was. Together with the

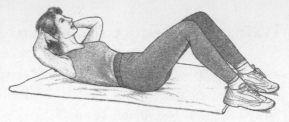

Figure 9: Abdominal Curl

back extension exercise, the abdominal curl (see figure 9) will improve the strength and stability of your torso while helping to flatten and trim your tummy.

Instructions

1. Lie on your back on a carpeted floor or mat with your knees bent and your feet flat on the floor. Place your hands behind your head and neck for support and keep your gaze toward the ceiling.
2. To a count of 3, slowly raise your head, neck, shoulders, and upper back off the floor, contracting your abdominal muscles.
3. Remember to breathe.
4. To minimize stress on your back, keep your head and neck in alignment, make sure to keep your gaze upward (not toward your knees), and lift your chest toward the ceiling.
5. Pause. Then, to a count of 3, slowly lower your body back down to the starting position.
6. On one of your first few abdominal curls, place one hand on your abdominal muscles and feel them contract; remember to move slowly and focus on using your abs (not your head or shoulders) to lift your body from the ground.
7. Complete 2 sets of 10 repetitions, with a break of approximately 1 minute between sets.

Balance Training to Reduce the Risk of Falls

Balance is essential to reducing your risk for falls and fractures. Yet as we age, our balance slowly deteriorates—unless we do something to maintain it. The poses below (see figures 10 and 11) will be familiar to you if you have ever taken a yoga class; they are simple but very effective as a means to improve balance in a short period of time.

MOUNTAIN POSE AND SWAY

1. Stand with your feet together, knees slightly bent, and arms at your sides.
2. Stand tall and straight with your shoulders down and relaxed.
3. Distribute your weight evenly throughout the heel, ball, and toes of your foot.

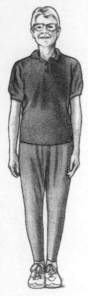

4. Starting with your feet, focus on how each region of your body is connected and in alignment—the sole of your foot with each foot and ankle stacked above; your shin bones, knees, and thighs side by side; your hips, ribs, and shoulders symmetrically stacked with arms hanging loosely at your sides; and your spine, neck, and head in gentle alignment.
5. Remember to breathe deeply. Remain in this position for 1 to 3 minutes.
6. Once you become comfortable in the mountain pose and you feel that your weight is equally distributed in both feet, slowly sway left, right, forward, and backward without moving your feet. Your hips and back should remain relaxed and stable, with only the slightest bend coming from your ankle. Continue this movement for 1 to 3 minutes.

Figure 10:
Mountain Pose
and Sway

7. If you feel unstable in this position at first, widen your stance. Practice the stance for a few minutes more, swaying regularly, and eventually bringing your feet together.

ONE-LEGGED STORK

1. Stand beside a sturdy table or counter with your feet shoulder-width apart, knees soft, and arms at your sides.
2. Bend one knee and rotate your hip and thigh outward, bringing the sole of your foot to the inner part of the standing leg.
3. Place the sole of your foot above or below—not directly on—your knee joint.
4. Be conscious of how your weight is distributed throughout your foot on the supporting leg; try to put the same amount of weight in your heel as in your toes.
5. Slowly raise your arms out to the side (or gently place one hand on the counter or table) to help maintain your balance, and gaze straight ahead.

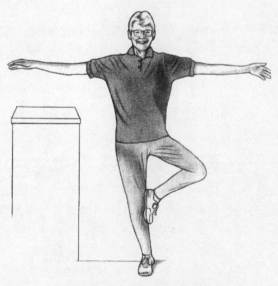

Figure 11: One-Legged Stork

6. Hold the position for 30 seconds to 2 minutes, lower your foot back to the ground, and then repeat on the other leg.

Flexibility Exercises for Healthy Joints and Muscles

Always follow any kind of strength training with flexibility exercises as part of your daily routines (see figures 12 through 15). Stretching will help your muscles stay limber and minimize soreness after lifting weights. For general health, stretching promotes relaxation and overall flexibility and reduces your risk for injuries.

QUADRICEPS STRETCH

To stretch the muscles of the front of your upper leg:

1. Stand with feet shoulder-width apart and knees soft in front of a sturdy chair.

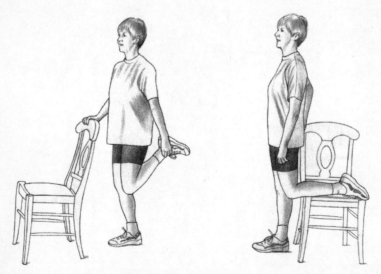

Figure 12: Quadriceps Stretch

2. Slowly bend your left knee, bring your foot behind your left buttock, and grasp your ankle with your left hand. Keep your thighs side by side and hold the position.
3. If you are unable to grasp your ankle behind you while keeping your thighs side by side, place your lower leg on the seat of a chair (as shown).
4. Breathe normally while holding the stretch for 20 to 30 seconds. Return to starting position, complete the stretch on the other leg, and repeat on both legs if desired.

HAMSTRING AND CALF STRETCH

To stretch the muscles of the back of your upper and lower leg:

1. Stand with feet shoulder-width apart and knees soft in front of a sturdy chair.
2. Slowly bend at the hip and, keeping a flat back, lower your hands to the seat of the chair.
3. Make sure not to round your back. Bend down only as far as the flexibility of your legs will allow while keeping your back straight and in alignment with your neck and head.
4. Breathe normally while holding the stretch for 20 to 30 seconds. Return to starting position and repeat if desired.

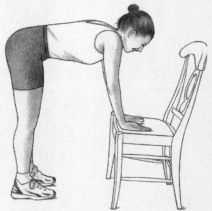

Figure 13: Hamstring and Calf Stretch

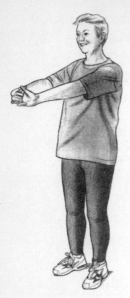

Figure 14:
Shoulder Stretch

SHOULDER STRETCH

To stretch the muscles of your arms, shoulders, and upper back:

1. Stand with feet shoulder-width apart and knees soft.
2. Lace your fingers together in front of you, and then rotate your wrists to face your palms away from your body.
3. Press your palms outward, raising your arms to chest height, and push through your hands so that you feel a stretch through your shoulders and upper back.
4. Breathe normally while holding the stretch for 20 to 30 seconds. Return to starting position and repeat if desired.

CHEST STRETCH

To stretch the muscles of your arms, shoulders, and chest:

1. Stand with feet shoulder-width apart and knees soft.
2. Grasp your hands behind your back, gently pulling them straight behind you as high as you can.
3. If you're unable to grasp your hands behind your back, use a facecloth or hand towel to bridge the gap; complete the stretch as if your hands were grasped. As your shoulder and chest flexibility

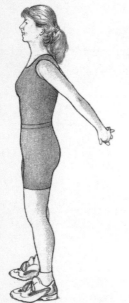

Figure 15: Chest Stretch

increases, you may be able to complete the stretch without using a cloth or towel.

4. Breathe normally while holding the stretch for 20 to 30 seconds. Return to starting position and repeat if desired.

Sample Exercise Programs

The following exercise programs are designed to be done three to five times a week. For the maximum benefit, you should try to spend 30 to 60 minutes *every day* engaging in a sport or leisure activity such as yoga, golf, or gardening. If you choose the three-day-a-week program, be sure to increase the amount of leisure activity you engage in.

FIVE-DAY PROGRAM

Daily: 30 to 60 minutes of sport or leisure activity (e.g., yoga or gardening)

Monday:
   30 minutes of brisk walking (or running if appropriate)
   4 Stretching exercises
   2 Balance-training exercises
Tuesday:
   7 Strength-training exercises
   4 Stretching exercises
Wednesday:
   30 minutes of stair climbing (or running if appropriate)
   4 Stretching exercises
   2 Balance-training exercises
Thursday:
   7 Strength-training exercises
   4 Stretching exercises

Friday:
   30 minutes of elliptical training (or running if appropriate)
   4 Stretching exercises

THREE-DAY PROGRAM

Daily: 30 to 60 minutes of sport or leisure activity (e.g., yoga or gardening)

Wednesday:
   30 minutes of brisk walking (or running if appropriate)
   4 Stretching exercises
   2 Balance-training exercises

Saturday:
   30 minutes of cycling (or running if appropriate)
   1–3 Strength-training exercises (lower body only)
   4 Stretching exercises

Sunday:
   30 minutes of elliptical training (or running if appropriate)
   4–7 Strength-training exercises (upper body and trunk only)
   4 Stretching exercises
   2 Balance-training exercises

7 Yoga for Healthy Bones

Linda Sparrowe
Yoga Sequences by Patricia Walden

Linda Sparrowe, former managing editor and current contributing editor of Yoga Journal, *has long been associated with the yoga community. She currently directs the yoga program at the Mind/Body Center of the San Francisco Bay Club, where she's created a comprehensive continuing education program for yoga teachers. Her books, with Patricia Walden, include* A Woman's Book of Yoga and Health: A Lifelong Guide to Wellness *(Shambhala Publications, 2002),* Yoga for Healthy Bones, *and* Yoga for Healthy Menstruation *(Shambhala Publications, 2004). She is also author and project manager for* Yoga: A Yoga Journal Book, *a coffee-table book that honors the history and beauty of yoga's physical form.*

Patricia Walden, who designed the yoga sequences, is one of America's foremost yoga teachers and, according to Time *magazine, "the best yoga teacher in the world." She is regularly featured in* Yoga Journal *and is also the instructor on the videotape series called* Yoga Journal's Yoga Practice Series, *which have sold well over a million copies. She travels and teaches yoga all over the world.*

. . .

When you were younger, you probably thought about your bones only when you knocked your shin against a chair leg or perhaps broke a bone—in other words, only when they hurt. And then you concentrated on relieving the pain as quickly as possible and got back to your daily routine. But now you are nearing or already in menopause, and suddenly your bones have become a major health issue. Bones are as important to your overall health as your liver or kidneys or nervous system and, for most women, keeping them healthy takes some work. But keeping your bones strong and healthy doesn't have to be unpleasant work, and yoga is a great way to relax and strengthen your bones at the same time.

Yoga is a practice that dates back more than two thousand years. Although there are many styles of yoga, the goal of each is to bring the body to a state of awareness and relaxation through a series of specific poses. Special emphasis is placed on slow, deep breathing during each pose and on proper body alignment. The poses vary from simple to complex, depending on the experience of the person. Many people who practice yoga report increased muscle strength, better flexibility and balance, decreased back pain, and an overall feeling of relaxation and well-being. While yoga is generally safe if practiced correctly, people with certain joint or muscle conditions or osteoporosis should consult a physician before beginning a yoga program.

A daily yoga practice—one that takes your body through its full range of motion—improves your posture and balance and tones your muscles, which reduces abnormal demand on your joints. Many poses also involve weight-bearing resistance, which increases bone mass. Regular practice can lead to a more restful sleep and can help reduce your stress level, which can contribute significantly to the health of your bones. Even if your aches and pains stem from a serious degenerative disorder such as osteoarthritis or osteoporosis, a consistent yoga practice, coupled with a sound diet and healthy lifestyle habits, can help stabilize your condition and improve quality of life. (For more on osteoporosis, see chapter 6.)

You can do very little about many of the risk factors for osteoporosis—they're genetic. If you are very thin with a small frame, for example, you fit the body profile with the highest risk for the disease. Quite simply, your bones aren't as strong and dense as those of a larger-boned woman or an average-sized man. However, there are a number of things you *can* do to protect your bones, such as not smoking, limiting your alcohol intake, adopting a healthy diet rich in green leafy vegetables and whole grains, and getting plenty of appropriate exercise (for more on risk factors, see chapter 6).

How Yoga Can Help

A consistent yoga practice can strengthen your bones and keep your adrenal glands healthy in order to produce the level of hormones you will need after menopause. On pages 195 to 211, we have provided a specially designed yoga sequence aimed at reversing or preventing bone loss. Its purpose is to take your body through its full range of motion using standing and balancing poses, back bends, forward bends, inversions, and other asanas (poses) to keep you flexible and strong.

Yoga eases general menopausal symptoms as well by balancing the endocrine system and smoothing out the hormonal changes that take place during the menopausal phase. For example, the posture shoulder stand has been valued for centuries for its cooling effect on the body, and women have used it to effectively counter the effects of hot flashes. Forward bends encourage surrender and acceptance of the physical changes that are taking place and promote relaxation. Yoga helps relax the mind and body and combats the emotional stresses of the menopausal transition.

Improving Your Posture with Yoga

Poor posture in your early years heightens the risk of developing hyperkyphosis (an excessive curvature of the upper part of the spine), which is a risk factor for osteoporotic fractures later in life. Hyperkyphosis is a common condition in elderly people that affects the spine from the base of the neck to the top of the lower back. Excessive curvature in the thoracic spine leads to the "hunched over" appearance. Hyperkyphosis usually is not painful but may restrict your ability to perform daily activities, such as standing from the seated position, reaching for objects, and bending over.

Some cases of hyperkyphosis are caused by vertebral fractures, and in those cases the spinal curvature is presumably irreversible. However, only about half of people with this condition have a history of a vertebral fracture. In many cases, the curvature may be due in part to poor posture or muscle weakness, factors that may be modified by doing yoga. According to a study in *American Journal of Public Health,* specific yoga poses that target the upper back appear to help straighten the spine and restore physical function.[1]

One manifestation of poor posture and/or weak muscles is the forward, jutting head position. People who work at computers or have sedentary lifestyles often adopt this postural misalignment. When you sit, stand, or walk with your head forward on your neck, your upper back and neck muscles tighten in an attempt to hold your head up. Chronically strained upper back and neck muscles can bring on tension headaches or even arthritis in that area. After a while, these same muscles may become overstretched and weakened from all that work, which can lead to intervertebral disk problems in your neck and eventual stress fractures.

You may think that this condition affects only your upper back and neck muscles, but jutting your head forward has consequences throughout your entire body. Remember that in order to bend, twist, and rotate properly, your spine must be aligned correctly; the vertebrae must stack; the cervical, thoracic, and lumbar spines must maintain their curves; and the supporting muscles must relax completely when they are not in use. When you have bad posture, your head moves out of alignment, your cervical curve (neck area) decreases, your thoracic curve (between the neck and the diaphragm) exaggerates, and your lumbar curve (back and sides between the lowest ribs and the pelvis) flattens. As your thoracic spine rounds, it compromises your ability to twist and rotate your upper back, which puts greater pressure on your lumbar spine to perform those functions.

Forward head position signals the brain that your muscles need help responding to stress, so your adrenal glands start producing cortisol, the stress hormone that triggers the fight-or-flight response. Your shoulder blades move out of alignment, causing rotator cuff problems and inflammation in the surrounding tissues. Your collarbones move forward; your chest collapses inward; and your lungs—lacking adequate space to function—press against your diaphragm, moving it downward against the abdominal wall. Your abdominal muscles weaken, which in turn causes more problems in your lumbar spine.

Unless you correct this chronic postural problem, it will only get worse. Yoga can help by addressing the emotional as well as the physical causes of poor posture. Yogis believe that we store much of our emotional pain in the solar plexus (the area between the heart and the navel); our instinctive desire to protect ourselves also comes from that area of the body. So, if you suffer from poor self-esteem or the "poor me" blues, you have what yogis call "a closed heart," and you try to create a protective barrier around it by rounding your shoulders and allowing your chest to cave inward. Any poses that open up the chest will open your heart and bring you joy. But to successfully counteract the rounded shoulders, compressed diaphragm, and protruding abdomen, you must strengthen your upper back muscles, too.

Standing poses aim to correct posture by concentrating on proper alignment and strengthening your core (in and around your navel); they also help to ground your energy. What that means in "non-yogic" terms is that whenever you inhale deeply and then exhale your attention out of your head and into your body you feel less flighty and more grounded. Shoulder and neck openers relax and release the muscles in those areas, allowing the life force (what the Chinese call qi and yogis call prana) to move toward the heart region. Back bends open the chest, which increases lung capacity and circulation, and strengthen the back muscles. Inversions rebalance the nervous system. A daily practice of poses (such as the sequence to reverse or prevent bone loss on pages 195 to 211) that flex, extend, and rotate your spine is ideal for promoting good posture.

Yoga Is the Perfect Exercise

Studies consistently show that exercise increases bone mass in postmenopausal women. It is important to exercise consistently—at least thirty minutes a day, five days a week. Exercise works because it stimulates bone remodeling and improves the absorption of calcium by the bones. Not just any kind of exercise will do, however. Weight-bearing exercises and movements that exert pressure on your bones are what stimulate them to retain calcium. Generally, health-care providers recommend walking or running because these exercises stimulate the bones in your feet, legs, pelvis, and spine by combining the effects of gravity and muscle contraction (for more on specific exercises for bone health, see chapter 6). In contrast, swimming (which can help ease joint pain and increase limited mobility) does nothing to increase bone density.

Yoga is a good choice for a weight-bearing exercise. For some people, it may be better than walking or running because with yoga there is less negative impact and yoga exerts pressure on all your bones, not just those in your lower body. If tests indicate that you've already begun to lose bone mass—and may therefore be susceptible to vertebral stress fractures—you should particularly avoid running, because it puts too much stress on your knees, ankles, and lumbar spine. You can continue (or start) practicing yoga, however, because you can modify the poses as needed without diminishing their effectiveness.

Handstands and full backbends challenge your fingers, hands, wrists, and shoulders to work together to hold up your body's weight. Headstand (Sirsasana) and Elbowstand (Pincha Mayurasana) stimulate the bones in your elbows and forearms, as well as those in your neck and spine. By taking your spine through its full range of motion, a complete yoga practice improves your posture and keeps the muscles surrounding your bones flexible and strong.

Yoga Can Open Your Lungs and Relax Your Body

Yoga postures strengthen and relax your chest and back muscles, expand your lungs to increase stamina and respiration, and calm the body. This is particularly beneficial for perimenopausal women who suffer from fatigue, low-grade depression, and fuzzy thinking. You'll reap the same benefits from doing a series of slow, deliberate yoga poses in which you breathe steadily and mindfully as you would from a brisk thirty-minute walk.

In addition to strengthening poses, a woman who is suffering from menopausal symptoms will want to add to her yoga practice poses that open up the chest and poses that calm anxiety. (The exercises mentioned here are also especially helpful for those who suffer from asthma or other lung-related conditions.) Standing poses and back bends energize the body and draw oxygen into your lungs. Forward bends combined with deep breathing calm and restore equilibrium. A yoga routine might include standing poses such as Mountain Pose (Tadasana), Triangle Pose (Trikonasana), and Half-Moon Pose (Ardha Chandrasana), as well as gentle, supported back bends like Bridge Pose (Setu Bandha Sarvangasana), Reclining Bound Angle Pose (Supta Baddha Konasana), and Camel Pose (Ustrasana). Use a chair for support, if necessary. Child's Pose (Adho Mukha Virasana) and Standing Forward Bend (Uttanasana) are relaxing poses that can be done on their own or in between other poses when you need a rest. Always complete your practice with five to ten minutes of Corpse Pose (Savasana).

Yoga and Smoking

As if there weren't enough reasons to quit, studies now show a strong correlation between poor bone health and cigarette smoking. A 1994 Australian study concluded that women who smoked one pack of cigarettes daily throughout adulthood would have a deficit of 5 to 10 percent in bone density by the time they reached menopause, which is enough to increase the risk of fractures. Researchers found a decrease in serum concentrations of parathyroid hormone (PTH) and calcium, as well as a greater amount of calcium excreted from the kidneys, an indication that calcium was being leached from the bones.[2]

Although researchers don't know for sure why cigarette smoking causes low bone density, one reason could be that smokers have a more difficult time absorbing nutrients from the foods they eat. Malabsorption of calcium, magnesium, vitamin D, and other vitamins and minerals from foods can cause the body to search for other suppliers, such as the bones. Also, cigarette smoking appears to lower the amount of estrogen in the bloodstream, and, since estrogen slows the bone-destroying abilities of osteoclasts, less estrogen means softer bones.

Yoga alone can't stop the urge for nicotine, but it can help. If a daily smoking habit calms your anxiety, try forward bends or supported inversions. Many women, after doing yoga consistently for several months, report that they no longer crave a cigarette. "Practicing yoga, even a few minutes of concentrated breathing, stopped me from reaching for that next cigarette," said Caroline, a magazine editor with a ten-year, pack-a-day habit.

Yoga and Depression

The latest research suggests that depression in premenopausal women is a significant risk factor for osteoporosis. In the book *Women's Bodies, Women's Wisdom,* Christiane Northrup estimates that at least a quarter of all women in the United States battle serious depression sometime in their lives.

Many women find depression to be incapacitating, especially when combined with other symptoms of menopause. They describe the feelings of depression as the world pressing down on them, a weight on their chest, shallow breathing, no desire to do anything. This is one type of depression; it grips your entire being and leaves you feeling empty. But thousands of women suffer from another, equally insidious type of depression that is marked by high levels of anxiety and is thus called anxiety-driven depression. Women with this kind of depression tend to be high-functioning and driven, but their high-stress lifestyle keeps them from experiencing the feelings beneath their tension and fear. They feel anxious all the time and find themselves easily agitated, quick to anger, and very impatient.

If you suffer from depression and have already begun a yoga or meditation practice, you know that all these emotions—sadness, despair, anxiety—affect more than your mental state. They manifest themselves in the body as menstrual irregularities, digestive disorders, and back or chest pain. Chronic depression or anxiety also takes its toll on your nervous system.

So, how does all this sadness and anxiety lead to brittle bones? If your depression relates to hormonal fluctuation (such as during perimenopause or menopause), a drop in estrogen levels could be the culprit. Too little estrogen has a negative effect on bone density, so hormonally charged depression could cause the body to build bone inefficiently. Both the thyroid and the parathyroid glands help regulate the amount of calcium in the bloodstream, so hypothyroidism—a condition that brings on both depression and fatigue—also upsets the way the body makes bone.

Elevated levels of the stress hormone cortisol appear to play a major role in depression-related osteoporosis. In a 1996 study funded by the National Institute of Mental Health (NIMH) and published in the *New England Journal of Medicine,* researchers found—among other indicators—higher than normal urinary cortisol levels in women with past or current depression.[3] High levels of cortisol, a hormone produced by the adrenal glands, may depress the body's ability to build bone. Although a new NIMH study is in the works to better understand the correlation between depression and bone loss, researchers now believe that cortisol plays a role, that depression impairs calcium absorption, and that other hormone deficiencies may contribute to low bone density.

Depression won't cause brittle bones on its own, of course. You have to have other risk factors as well—small frame, low peak bone mass, lack of ovulation, or you smoke or drink excessively. But the NIMH study's findings that the decrease in bone density was significant in twenty-four otherwise healthy premenopausal women (more than 13 percent at the neck; some 11 percent at the hip) suggest that depression-related bone loss could increase the lifetime risk of fracture by as much as 50 percent.

It's impossible to separate the physiological benefits of yoga from the emotional and spiritual ones. Patricia Walden says, "Thoughts affect feelings, which in turn affect physiology." By adopting a yoga practice, you may be able to reverse this trend and change your emotions by changing your physiology. For example, Inverted Staff Pose (Viparita Dandasana) is a back-bending chest opener. The simple act of lifting your chest can elevate your emotions and clear your mind. It creates space for your breath to move more freely, and freer breath brings lighter feelings. Back bends further release any blockage in and around your heart that could be contributing to your rounded shoulders and sunken chest.

Seated forward bends, on the other hand, can quiet a nervous system that goes into overdrive when you become anxious or fearful. This pose provides an invaluable antidote to cortisol overload. Inversions allow oxygenated blood to circulate more freely, which soothes and then energizes the glands in and around your head and throat. Standing poses can also elevate your mood, making you feel stronger and more capable (literally, "standing on your own two feet").

Corpse Pose (Savasana) and other restorative poses provide conscious rest for your sympathetic nervous system—and your whole body—so healing can take place. They induce a state of complete relaxation, so your brain can restore itself and rebalance its neurotransmitters.

Yoga reminds you that nothing is permanent, that you are not your feelings. By staying aware in a pose, especially one that challenges you at first, you learn that you can be uncomfortable, even unhappy, and still be all right. As your proficiency increases, you come to see that what was impossible last week is doable today.

Working with your breath in the physical poses and during breathing practice (pranayama) can be a wonderful aid. Patricia says that deep, healing inhalations lift your spirits and that long, slow exhalations soothe your nerves. Don't be surprised if feelings of sadness, anger, or even fear well up inside you during your practice. Acknowledge these feelings and then let them go. They've been waiting to get out for a long time.

Do the practice in this chapter as often as your schedule allows. But try to do at least something every day—10 minutes of Corpse Pose (Savasana), for example—in order to lift your spirit and counteract the effects your moods have on your body.

A Yoga Sequence for Healthy Bones

Here is an easy-to-follow yoga sequence by Patricia Walden that is designed especially for perimenopausal and menopausal women to strengthen bones and muscles and promote relaxation.

- Mountain Pose (Tadasana) with different arm positions
- Standing Forward Bend (Uttanasana)
- Downward-Facing Dog Pose (Adho Mukha Svanasana)
- Warrior I Pose (Virabhadrasana I) and modifications
- Warrior II Pose (Virabhadrasana II) and modifications
- Extended Triangle Pose (Utthita Trikonasana) and modifications
- Revolved Triangle Pose (Parivrtta Trikonasana) and modifications
- Standing Spinal Twist Pose (Utthita Marichyasana)
- Camel Pose (Ustrasana)
- Child's Pose (Adho Mukha Virasana)
- Legs-Up-the-Wall Pose (Viparita Karani) and Legs-Up-the-Wall Cycle
- Corpse Pose (Savasana)

MOUNTAIN POSE (TADASANA)

Stand up straight, your legs together (with big toes touching, if that's comfortable; if not, keep your feet a few inches apart). Distribute your weight evenly between the front of your feet and your heels. Tighten your knees by pulling up with your quadriceps (front thigh muscles). Raise your sternum (breastbone) and broaden your chest by rolling your shoulders back and drawing your shoulder blades in. Lift your abdomen up and draw your tailbone in without pushing your thighs forward. Extend your arms downward with palms facing your thighs and fingers together (see figure 16A). Keep your shoulders moving away from your ears. Visualize your spine elongating, rising out of your center, as you plant your feet firmly on the ground. Breathe normally, relax your pelvic floor muscles (the ones you contract to stop urinating), shoulders, and neck. Remain in the pose for 30 to 60 seconds. Next, try the following variations on mountain pose.

ARMS OVERHEAD (URDHVA HASTASANA)

Standing in Mountain Pose (Tadasana), turn your palms outward and slowly lift your arms to the side and over your head, keeping your shoulders down and away from your ears (see figure 16B). Lift your chest and draw your shoulder blades deep into your back. (If you have trouble with balance, you may step your feet apart a little or practice with your back against a wall.) Stay in this pose for 20 to 30 seconds, if possible. Otherwise, come in and out two or three times.

ARMS IN PRAYER POSITION (NAMASKAR ARMS)

To further open your chest and shoulder area, continue standing in Mountain Pose (Tadasana), put your hands together in prayer position behind your back (see figure 16C). Be careful not to arch your back. If that's too much of a stretch, cross your arms behind you, holding your elbows (see figure 16D). Your posture should remain in alignment, just as it is when you have your arms by your sides.

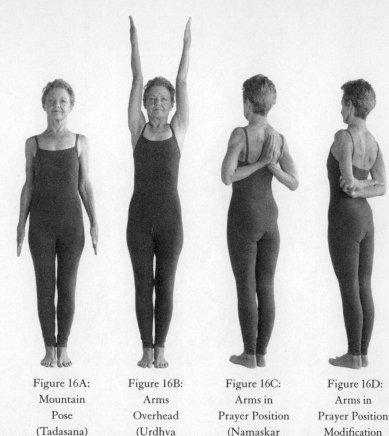

Figure 16A:
Mountain
Pose
(Tadasana)

Figure 16B:
Arms
Overhead
(Urdhva
Hastasana)

Figure 16C:
Arms in
Prayer Position
(Namaskar
Arms)

Figure 16D:
Arms in
Prayer Position
Modification

EFFECTS: The different arm positions help alleviate stiffness in your shoulders, arms, and upper and lower back; improve circulation throughout your body; and correct postural problems.

STANDING FORWARD BEND (UTTANASANA)

Begin this exercise (see figure 17) by standing with your feet slightly apart. Clasp your hands behind your back and, as you exhale, lengthen your waist and side ribs toward the floor. Bend forward. Keeping your hands clasped, extend through your arms and bring your hands overhead toward the floor. Keep your shoulder blades moving away from

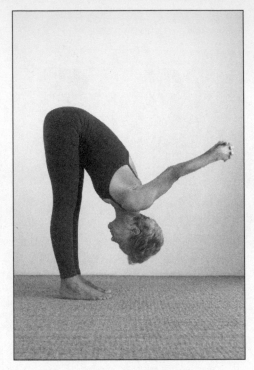

Figure 17: Standing Forward Bend
(Uttanasana)

your neck. Remain in this position for 10 to 15 seconds, slowly coming back to a standing position, and resting for a few breaths.

EFFECTS: By clasping your hands behind your back, you open your chest more and release tension and stiffness in your shoulders, elbows, wrists, and fingers.

DOWNWARD-FACING DOG POSE (ADHO MUKHA SVANASANA)

To find the correct distance between your hands and feet for this pose, lie facedown. Place your palms on the floor by each side of your chest with your fingers spread apart and pointing toward your head. Turn your toes inward. Come up on your hands and knees. (If you are flexible enough, keep your feet close together.) Exhale, press your hands into the mat, and

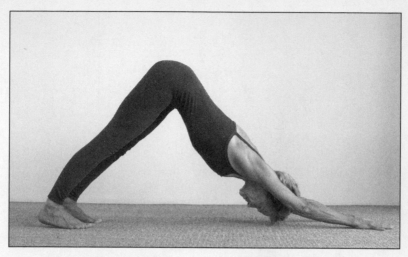

Figure 18: Downward-Facing Dog Pose (Adho Mukha Svanasana)

extend up through your inner arms. Exhale again and raise your buttocks high into the air (see figure 18). Move your thighs up and back, keep stretching through your legs, and bring your heels toward the floor as you lift your buttocks higher. The action of the arms and legs serves to elongate the spine and release your head. Stay in this pose for 30 seconds to 1 minute, breathing deeply. Let your head rest completely and release the base of your neck. To come out of the pose, return to your hands and knees, sit back on your heels, and slowly lift your head up.

EFFECTS: This weight-bearing exercise strengthens your arms, legs, and spine; helps elongate your spine; and eases tension and stiffness in your shoulders, neck, and arms.

WARRIOR I POSE (VIRABHADRASANA I)

Stand in Mountain Pose (Tadasana). Step your feet as far apart as is comfortable (about 4½ feet) with your toes pointing forward. Stretch your arms out to the sides at shoulder level, parallel to the floor, with palms down. Turn your palms up and raise both arms until they are in line with your ears and parallel to each other; your elbows should be straight (see

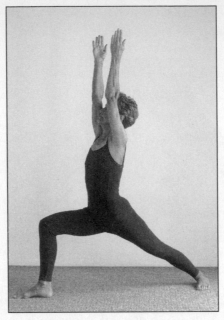

Figure 19: Warrior I Pose
(Virabhadrasana I)

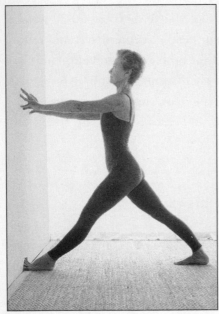

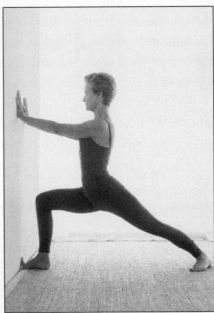

Figure 20: Warrior I Pose Modification A   Figure 21: Warrior I Pose Modification B

figure 19). Draw up through your quadriceps and lift your abdomen and chest. As you exhale, simultaneously turn your torso and right leg 90 degrees to the right and your left foot about 60 degrees to the right. (You should now be facing forward over your right leg. Try to keep your back [left] foot on the ground. But if this is too difficult, lift your heel off the ground.) Inhale and stretch through your upper arms; exhale and bend your right knee so your thigh and shin form a right angle. (If your knee extends beyond your ankle, you need to widen your stance.) Stretch your torso up toward the ceiling as you take your head back as far as it is comfortable and look up at your thumbs. (If this is too hard on your neck, keep your head straight and your gaze forward.) Move in and out of the pose several times by bending and straightening your right leg to create mobility in your hips and knees. Return to Mountain Pose (Tadasana) and switch legs.

MODIFICATION: If you need additional support or stability, press the toes of your front foot into the wall and place your hands on the wall in front of you. Look straight ahead (see figure 20). Move in and out of the pose with each exhalation, bending and straightening your front leg three or four times. Remember not to let your knee extend beyond your ankle (see figure 21). Breathe normally for several breaths.

EFFECTS: This weight-bearing pose helps increase mobility in your hips and lower back. Moving in and out of the pose helps keep your joints flexible.

WARRIOR II POSE (VIRABHADRASANA II)

Stand in Mountain Pose (Tadasana). Step your feet out as wide as possible (about 4½ feet apart, if you can); turn your left foot out 90 degrees and your right foot slightly inward. The heel of your left foot should line up with the arch of your right. Stretch your arms out to the sides so they're parallel to the floor (see figure 22). As you exhale, bend your left knee so your thigh is parallel and your shin is perpendicular to the floor. (If your knee extends beyond your ankle, you need to widen your stance.) Turn

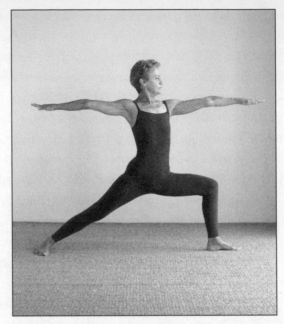

Figure 22: Warrior II Pose (Virabhadrasana II)

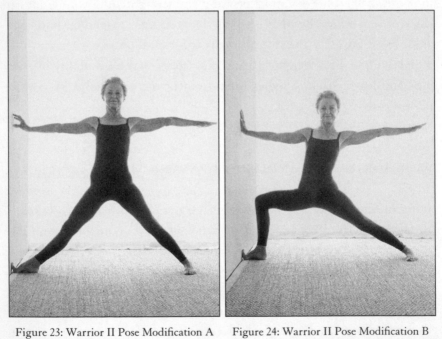

Figure 23: Warrior II Pose Modification A   Figure 24: Warrior II Pose Modification B

your head to look over your left arm just past your fingertips. Imagine both arms are engaged in a tug-of-war. Remain in the pose for several breaths or 15 to 20 seconds. Move in and out of the pose several times slowly to increase mobility in your joints. Step your feet together and change sides.

MODIFICATIONS: (A) If you need support, practice with one foot pressed up against a wall and your hand resting on it (see figure 23). (B) Move in and out of the pose by straightening as you inhale and bending the knee of the leg closest to the wall as you exhale, releasing your arms slightly if needed (see figure 24). As you come into the pose for the last time, remove your hand from the wall and remain in the pose for several breaths.

EFFECTS: This pose is great for improving posture; elongating and strengthening your spine; and increasing flexibility in your hips, back, and legs. Because it is a weight-bearing exercise for your feet, ankles, and legs, it stimulates the bones in those areas to retain calcium.

EXTENDED TRIANGLE POSE (UTTHITA TRIKONASANA)

Stand in Mountain Pose (Tadasana). Step your feet about 3½ feet apart; turn your right foot out 90 degrees and your left foot slightly inward. The heel of your right foot should line up with the arch of your left (see figure 25). Place a block beside the outside edge of your right foot. Stretch your arms out to the sides, draw up through your quadriceps, and lift your abdomen and chest. On an exhalation, keeping your back straight, extend your trunk to the right, and bring your right hand down to the block. Press your hand into the block, stretch across your chest and up through your left arm. Draw your shoulder blades in, turn your chest toward the ceiling, and look straight ahead or up at your left hand. Turn your abdomen to the left. Breathe normally and hold this pose for 20 to 30 seconds. On an inhalation, lift up and straighten your torso. Repeat the pose on your left side, then turn your toes forward and step your feet back toward each other, returning to Mountain Pose.

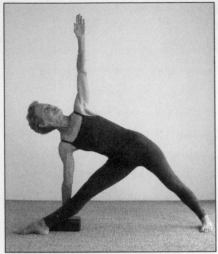

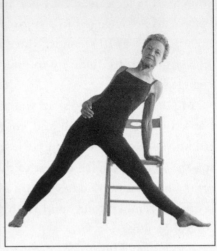

Figure 25: Extended Triangle Pose
(Utthita Trikonasana)

Figure 26: Extended Triangle Pose
Modification

MODIFICATION: If this pose proves too challenging or if you feel unsteady, substitute a low stool or chair for the block (see figure 26). Place one hand on the chair and another on your hip. Keep your arms and legs active and strong. Relax your shoulders, neck, and facial muscles and breathe normally for several breaths.

EFFECTS: This pose elongates and strengthens your spine and increases circulation to your pelvic region. It is excellent for helping increase flexibility and stability. Because it is a weight-bearing exercise for your arms, legs, and spine, it stimulates the bones in those areas to retain calcium.

REVOLVED TRIANGLE POSE (PARIVRTTA TRIKONASANA)

Stand in Mountain Pose (Tadasana). Step your feet about 3 to 3½ feet apart; turn your left foot out 90 degrees and your right foot slightly inward. The heel of your right foot should line up with the arch of your left (see figure 27). Place a block parallel to the outside edge of your left foot. As you exhale, rotate your torso so you are facing left; your right leg and knee should turn inward. Place the fingertips of your right hand on the block.

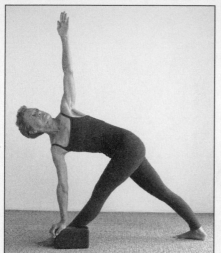

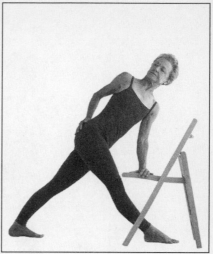

Figure 27: Revolved Triangle Pose
(Parivrtta Trikonasana)

Figure 28: Revolved Triangle Pose
Modification

Tighten both legs and keep your chest expanded by drawing your right shoulder blade into your back. Breathe normally for 15 to 20 seconds. Come up on an inhalation, turn, and repeat the pose on the other side.

MODIFICATION: If this pose is too difficult, place your hand on a chair instead of a block (see figure 28). If necessary, add blankets and bolsters to the chair to raise the height. Come in and out of the pose several times to keep your joints fluid and flexible. Hold the final pose for several breaths, if possible.

EFFECTS: This pose stimulates the bones in your legs, arms, and spine to retain calcium. It also elongates and strengthens your thoracic spine; increases flexibility and mobility in your shoulders, hips, and back; and improves your posture.

STANDING SPINAL TWIST POSE (UTTHITA MARICHYASANA)

Place a chair with one side against the wall and put a block on the seat area closest to the wall (see figure 29). If the block slips, place a sticky mat on the chair seat first. Stand facing the chair with the left side of

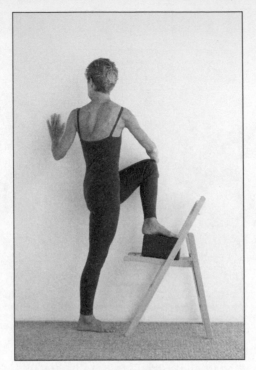

Figure 29: Standing Spinal Twist Pose
(Utthita Marichyasana)

your body next to the wall. Keeping your right leg firm, put your left foot up on the block. Inhale and stretch up, then exhale and turn your torso toward the wall, using your right hand on your left knee and your left hand on the wall. Move in and out of this pose several times, each time taking a deeper inhalation to stretch up taller and exhaling more completely to turn your torso a little more. Turn the chair and repeat with your right foot.

EFFECTS: This pose helps elongate and strengthen your spine and release stiffness in your upper and middle back.

CAMEL POSE (USTRASANA)

Kneel on the floor with your knees and feet hip-width apart. Place your palms on your buttocks and, as you exhale, move your thighs slightly for-

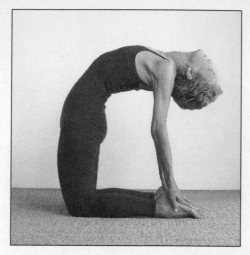

Figure 30: Camel Pose (Ustrasana)

ward and raise your side ribs. Gradually bend back as far as possible, lift your chest, and broaden your shoulders. Move your hands from your buttocks to your feet and take hold of your heels (see figure 30). If you can't reach your heels, place your hands on a chair positioned behind you, fingers pointing away from your body as much as possible. Your thighs should be perpendicular to the floor. Take your head back, if that's comfortable, and breathe steadily for 10 to 15 seconds. If that's too difficult at first, come into and out of the pose a few times. To come out, release your hands one at a time. As you exhale, slowly lift from your sternum, using your thigh muscles. Your head should come up last.

EFFECTS: This pose opens your chest, helps you breathe, increases energy, and promotes a sense of accomplishment. It has the added benefits of stimulating your vertebrae to retain calcium and building a strong spine and upper back muscles.

CHILD'S POSE (ADHO MUKHA VIRASANA)

Kneel on the floor with your knees slightly wider than your hips and bring your big toes together, if possible. Bend forward and stretch your

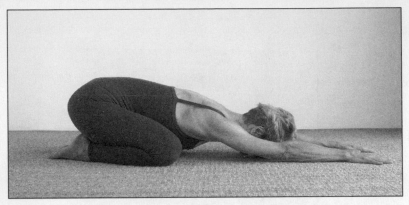

Figure 31: Child's Pose (Adho Mukha Virasana)

arms and trunk forward (see figure 31). Rest your head on the floor or on a blanket. Remain in this pose for 20 to 30 seconds (or more), moving your shoulder blades into your back ribs and elongating the back of your neck. To come up, press your hands into the floor and slowly sit up, lifting your head up last.

EFFECTS: This pose stretches and tones your entire spine while releasing the muscles in your neck and upper back. This pose also stretches out your back after backbends and helps calm your nerves.

LEGS-UP-THE-WALL (VIPARITA KARANI)

Place a bolster about 3 inches from the wall. Sit on the bolster so that your right hip and side are touching the wall. Using your hands to support you, lean back and swivel your body around as you take your right leg and then your left leg up the wall. Keep your buttocks close to or against the wall. (If you feel stiffness or discomfort in your legs, push your buttocks slightly away from the wall.) Lie down so that your lower back and ribs are supported by the bolster and your shoulders and head are on the floor. (If your neck is uncomfortable, put a folded towel or blanket under it.) Extend through your legs and place your arms above your head, elbows bent and palms up. Rest in this position, eyes closed, for at least 5 to 10 minutes (see figure 32).

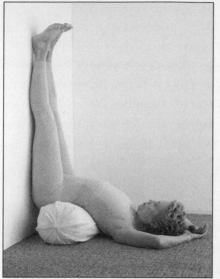

Figure 32: Legs-Up-the-Wall (Viparita Karami)

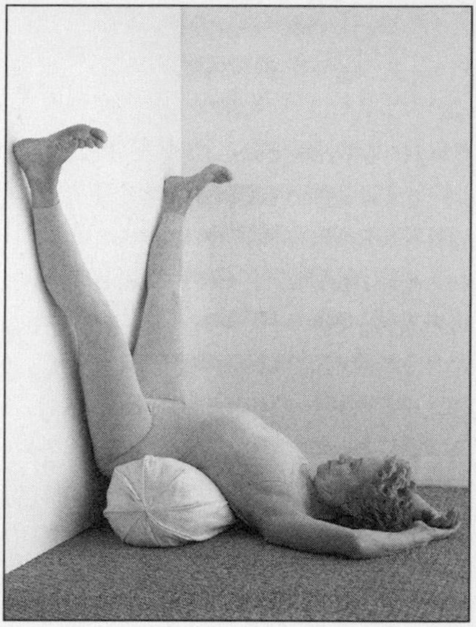

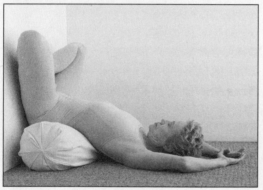

Figure 33: Legs-Up-the-Wall Cycle

Figure 34: Legs-Up-the-Wall Cycle

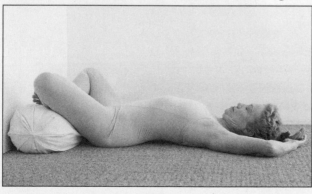

Figure 35: Legs-
Up-the-Wall Cycle

Legs-Up-the-Wall Cycle

Without moving your torso, allow your legs to open out to the sides (see figure 33). Remain in this position, breathing normally, for 3 to 5 minutes. Again, keeping your torso in the same position, bend your knees, cross your ankles, and continue in the pose for another 3 to 5 minutes (see figure 34). Then gently push away until your buttocks is just off the bolster and the tops of your thighs and legs remain on the bolster (see figure 35). Remain resting in this position for 3 to 5 minutes, or as long as you like. To come out of the pose, uncross your legs, push gently away from the bolster, and roll to one side. Breathe quietly there for a few breaths and then use your arms to help you to a seated position.

EFFECTS: This pose relieves nervous exhaustion and helps balance your nervous system, mitigating the effects of stress hormones (cortisol and adrenaline).

CORPSE POSE (SAVASANA)

Lie on the floor with a blanket under your head and neck (if desired), and stretch your legs out in front of you (see figure 36). Place your arms comfortably at your sides, slightly away from your torso, with your palms facing the ceiling. Actively stretch your arms and legs away from

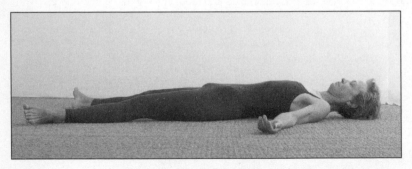

Figure 36: Corpse Pose (Savasana)

you and then allow them to release completely. Close your eyes and let everything relax. Take a few deep breaths, inhaling the breath into your chest without tensing the throat, neck, or diaphragm. Exhale your body into the mat, releasing your shoulders, neck, and facial muscles. Keep the abdomen soft and relaxed and release the lower back. As your eyes relax back into the sockets, begin to breathe normally for at least 5 to 10 minutes. To come out of the pose, bend your knees, roll slowly to one side, and, after a few breaths, gently push yourself to a seated position.

EFFECTS: A wonderfully resting pose, Savasana deeply relaxes and soothes the sympathetic nervous system, relieves fatigue and anxiety, and restores balance.

8 Managing Incontinence and the Overactive Bladder

Janis Luft, R.N., N.P., MSN

Janis Luft is a women's health nurse-practitioner at the University of California, San Francisco (UCSF), Department of Obstetrics/Gynecology and Reproductive Sciences, and an assistant clinical professor in the Department of Family Health, UCSF School of Nursing. In addition, she is a research nurse-practitioner with the UCSF Women's Health Clinical Research Center. She received her bachelor of science degree in nursing from the University of Pennsylvania and her master of science degree in nursing from the Ambulatory Women's Health Care Nurse-Practitioner Program at UCSF. Luft designed and coordinates the Pelvic Floor Rehabilitation and Behavioral Training Program at the UCSF Women's Continence Center. The author of several journal articles, book chapters, and abstracts on the subject of urinary incontinence, she has lectured extensively on the subject. She is currently an editorial reviewer for Geriatric Nursing.

At age fifty-five, Barbara was considering retiring. She'd always loved her career as a teacher at a busy community college and found it personally rewarding. But her daily teaching schedule was very full, and lately it was becoming increasingly difficult to get through her entire two-hour seminar without a bathroom break. About halfway through, she'd start to get that uncomfortable feeling of being overly full in the bladder. Waiting too long could produce disastrous results. Recently, she'd rushed out at the end of a class, leaving students with questions in her dust, barely making it to the ladies' room half a hallway away, only to find all the stalls occupied. And then it happened: she actually had an accident because she just couldn't wait any longer. Even though she'd tried to ignore it, the problem that had been nagging at her for a couple of years had gotten worse and worse, especially over the past six months. She had started limiting the amount of liquid she drank during the day and slipping into the bathroom as often as she could, but even these precautions weren't working anymore. The thought of having another accident while she was at school was mortifying. Though she'd really wanted to continue teaching for a few more years, the risk of losing control in class was more than she could bear. Early retirement seemed to be the only answer.

Bladders Behaving Badly

By the age of sixty-five, about half of all women will have some problem with urinary incontinence (UI), the involuntary loss of urine. Although young women are not immune either—about one in four reproductive-age women report experiencing incontinence—for them, bladder problems are usually transient (for example, occurring during or shortly after pregnancy and eventually resolving). About 18 million Americans suffer from incontinence, and approximately 85 percent are women. Pregnancy and childbirth, menopause, and the structure of the female urinary tract account for the difference in numbers of women versus men with this condition. But older women—those over fifty—are the most likely to suffer from incontinence problems.

According to best estimates, upward of $32 billion a year is spent on the problem of incontinence, *more than is spent on the care of women suffering from all forms of cancer!* And unfortunately, more than 75 percent of this cost is borne by the very women suffering from the problem.[1] Visits to health-care providers, prescription medication, and surgery account for much of this cost, but a significant amount is due to the purchase of hygiene products (pads, adult diapers, disposable undergarments) and the extra cleaning costs (clothing and furniture) necessitated by wetting accidents. These latter costs are largely borne by the consumer, as most insurers and Medicare do not pay for incontinence products.

Sadly, women may not perceive loss of bladder control as a health problem, but rather as an inevitable part of aging. While it is true that bladder problems become more common as we grow older, urinary incontinence is *not* a normal part of aging. The misperception that this is "just what happens" or embarrassment often discourages women from speaking out and seeking help. And health-care providers often fail to ask about issues of bladder control. Urinary incontinence is truly a "don't ask, don't tell" health-care issue. A survey of more than 45,000 American households published in 2003 reported that of the 1,970 women who acknowledged symptoms of urinary incontinence on a questionnaire, less than half had spoken to a health-care provider about the problem.[2] But incontinence is a treatable condition. And as researchers learn more about the causes of UI, it may also become a preventable condition.

UI is more than just an inconvenience. It can severely decrease an individual's quality of life. Fear of leakage or accidents can and does cause embarrassment and social isolation.[3] A woman who worries about wetness and odor may refrain from exercising, spending time with family or friends, traveling—in short, all the things that make life worth living. Urge urinary incontinence (also called overactive bladder [OAB]) in the elderly increases the likelihood of hip fractures or other broken bones, since getting up at night to urinate is a major cause of falling.[4] Overactive bladder has also been shown to be highly associated with increased urinary tract infections, skin irritation and infection, and depression.[5]

Bladder Problems and Menopause

Many experts believe that menopause is a major risk factor for both stress and urge incontinence. UI is a more common problem as women age, and midlife appears to be a time that women frequently begin to notice problems with bladder control. In addition, the urinary tract develops from the same embryologic structures that form the genital tract. Like the vulva, vagina, and uterus, the bladder, urethra, and ureters are rich in estrogen receptors. The loss of estrogen production that characterizes menopause results in anatomic and physiologic changes to the female urinary tract. This includes thinning of the mucous layer that lines the urethra, a decrease in the closure pressure of the urethra, and a lowered sensory threshold in the bladder. These changes are thought to contribute to bladder muscle weakness, which in turn increases susceptibility to incontinence.

However, medical research has failed to establish a direct link between menopause and the development of incontinence. Despite the lack of evidence of a connection between menopause and incontinence, the fact is that the incidence of UI increases with age. Epidemiologists who reviewed thirteen studies that tried to define the prevalence of female UI found that 20 to 30 percent of women in young adult life had some degree of urine leakage, which increased to 30 to 40 percent around middle age, and then increased again in the elderly (ranging from 30 to 50 percent in different studies).[6]

Because incontinence is such a major issue for women of a certain age and because these same women are often suffering from menopause as well, we feel that it is crucial to include a chapter on this very important health complaint in this book on menopause.

The Basics of Normal Bladder Function

Your bladder (and mine, for that matter) has two simple functions: to store and expel urine. Simply put, women with UI are great at expelling but lousy at storing.

The bladder is located within the pelvis, tucked between the pubic bone (in front) and uterus and intestines (behind and above). Two long, thin tubes called ureters insert into the dome of the bladder on either side. They carry urine produced in the kidneys to the bladder, which fills passively. The bladder itself is composed mostly of smooth muscle, the same type that makes up your intestines and lungs. The medical term for this balloon-shaped muscle is detrusor.

Urine exits the bladder through the urethra, a two-inch tube made of both smooth muscle (the type in your lungs and intestines) and striated muscle (the same type in your biceps and other voluntary muscles). The urethra is lined with mucous-producing tissues that fold together to help seal the urethra and keep urine in the bladder. The urethra passes through a large band of muscles, which create the "pelvic floor" (PF), called the levator ani complex. These muscles extend front to back from

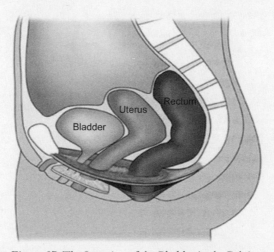

Figure 37: The Location of the Bladder in the Pelvis

the symphysis pubis (pubic bone) to the coccyx (tailbone) and attach on the sides to the walls of the pelvis. The vagina and the anus also pass through small openings in the PF muscles. In their resting state, the PF muscles remain a bit taut, creating a sphincter effect. It is the combination of the PF muscles, the musculature of the urethra itself, and its mucosal lining that maintains urethral pressure—essential to keeping urine in the bladder until the need and socially acceptable opportunity to expel it arise.

The bladder can hold about ten to twenty ounces when we are young adults; however, this capacity declines as we age. On average, most young women urinate about every four to six hours. Urinating eight or fewer times a day is considered normal. By the age of sixty-five, urinating every three to four hours and waking up at night once or twice may be normal. As it fills with urine, the bladder expands to accommodate the increasing volume without any appreciable increase in pressure within the bladder itself. During storage, the pressure in the urethra is always higher than the pressure within the bladder. This is how we keep urine in until we are ready to let it out. When we *are* ready to go, we (usually) sit, the PF muscles relax, and this is followed immediately by a bladder (detrusor) contraction. Voilà—urination!

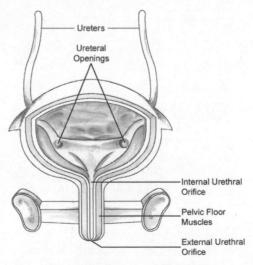

Figure 38: The Urinary Bladder

When we are born, urinating is an "involuntary" activity: bladder fills, bladder empties. Our "micturition center" is located in the spinal cord, and when the stretch receptors in the bladder wall signal sufficient fullness, the center sends a message for the bladder to contract. But as our brain and muscle control develop and our parents' patience with diaper changing wears thin, we learn bladder socialization, otherwise known as "potty training." We literally train the thinking part of our brains, the cerebral cortex, to stop the bladder from contracting until we are in the appropriate setting.

As the bladder fills, the stretch receptors within the bladder walls send our brains "fullness" signals, which increase in volume as we near our threshold capacity. The micturition center in the cerebral cortex inhibits bladder contraction until we decide that it is "time to go." Then the signals for the PF muscles to relax and the bladder to contract are carried through the spine and to the appropriate end organs via the pudendal and sacral nerves. They exit the spinal column in the lower spine. The bladder receives the message to contract with the help of a neurochemical called acetylcholine. Other neurochemicals relay the message of relaxation to the PF muscles. (Later in the chapter, when we discuss indications used to treat incontinence, this information will become more important.)

The Abnormal Bladder

Urinary incontinence can, at times, be an acute problem; that is, occurring suddenly and unexpectedly. In older women, acute UI can be a symptom of a urinary tract infection (UTI). In our younger years, the principal symptoms of a UTI or bladder infection are an increase in the frequency and urgency of urination and pain or burning with urination. However, the elderly bladder may no longer be able to sense the bladder wall irritation that infection can cause. But bacterial buildup within the bladder and the toxins produced by UTI can cause the pressure within the urethra to weaken. Lower-than-normal urethral pressure increases the likelihood of leakage.

Certain medications that are prescribed for other conditions can increase the risk of acute UI. Check with your health-care provider if you have recently started a new medication and have noticed an increasing problem with bladder control. Below is a list of medications that may affect bladder function.

Medications That May Affect Bladder Function

Type of Medication	Common Names	Possible Side Effects
Antidepressants, antipsychotics, sedatives/hypnotics	Elavil, Tofranil, Haldol, Valium	Drowsiness, retention
Diuretics (water pills)	Maxide, Diazide	Frequency, urgency
Caffeine		Frequency, urgency
Anticholinergics	ProBanthine	Retention
Narcotics	Morphine, Demerol, Percocet	Retention, constipation, drowsiness
Alpha-adrenergic blockers	Cardura, Minipress, Hytrin	Decreased urethral pressure
Alpha-adrenergic agonists	Sudafed, Phenylpropanolamine	Increased urethral pressure, retention
Beta-adrenergic agonists	Epinephrine, Theophylline, Albuterol	Inhibited bladder function, retention
Calcium channel blockers	Calan, Procardia, Cardizem	Retention
ACE inhibitors	Accupril, Lotensin, Vasotec	Chronic cough
Selective serotonin reuptake inhibitors (SSRIs)	Prozac, Paxil, Zoloft, Lexapro	Frequency, urgency, retention

By far the largest percentage of women with bladder control problems have chronic incontinence. Many women have symptoms that slowly worsen over a period of years, but they do nothing about it until the symptoms are unbearable. As their bladder begins to dictate more of their life and consumes more personal and financial resources, these women may finally resolve to speak to a health-care provider about the problem. If you think you are experiencing signs of urinary incontinence, it's important to understand what it is, why it is happening (if possible), and what your treatment options are.

Types of Incontinence

STRESS URINARY INCONTINENCE

Stress urinary incontinence (SUI) is a medical condition in which involuntary loss of urine occurs during physical activity such as coughing, sneezing, laughing, or exercise—especially impact exercises—and lifting. In more severe cases, simply standing up from a sitting position or stepping off a curb may cause a leak. *Stress* in this context refers to pressure on the bladder. Risk factors for stress incontinence include being a woman, advanced age, childbirth, smoking, and obesity. Conditions that cause chronic coughing, such as chronic bronchitis and asthma, may also increase the risk of stress incontinence.

In a normal bladder, the urethra remains in its normal anatomical position, allowing the pressure from the top of the bladder to be transmitted along the urethra equally on all sides. At the same time, the muscles of the pelvic floor that hug the urethra tighten slightly to ensure that the urethra stays closed. When the urethra sags and fails to maintain internal pressure, a leakage can occur. Likewise the pelvic muscles may fail to respond quickly enough or with sufficient force to keep the urethra closed.

URGE URINARY INCONTINENCE (UUI)
OR OVERACTIVE BLADDER (OAB)

Urge urinary incontinence (UUI) is a condition in which you experience a sudden or mounting sense of urgency to urinate caused by involuntary bladder contractions. These involuntary contractions of the bladder, which often occur at inappropriate times, can be random or triggered by an outside stimulus such as the sound of running water.

UUI is the most common type of incontinence in women over the age of sixty.[7] It is estimated that 60 to 70 percent of urinary incontinence in this age group is due to UUI. Women with urge incontinence report losing small or large amounts of urine because "I just couldn't make it to the bathroom fast enough." This can occur even when the bladder is not particularly full. Women with urge urinary incontinence also typically complain of frequent urination and having to get out of bed several times a night to urinate (nocturia).

The term *overactive bladder (OAB)* is often used for urge incontinence. In a general sense, overactive bladder describes the conditions of urinary frequency, urgency, and nighttime urination. Leaking accidents may be avoided by carefully regulating fluid intake, making frequent trips to the bathroom, and carefully planning errands around the availability of public facilities. Sleep is disrupted. As the problem progresses, the sufferer may limit social activities or make lifestyle changes in order to remain closer to the bathroom.

Although the causes of UUI or OAB are largely unknown, it is thought that dysfunction of the nerves controlling the bladder may be a factor. Other bladder injuries, such as diverticula or stones, might also be factors.

OVERFLOW URINARY INCONTINENCE (OUI)

Overflow urinary incontinence usually occurs in older women or severe diabetics whose bladders do not contract forcefully enough to expel urine. Although it is less common in women, OUI can be caused by conditions that obstruct the bladder. In some cases, severe constipation can obstruct the flow of urine, resulting in temporary overflow incontinence.

FUNCTIONAL URINARY INCONTINENCE

The term *functional urinary incontinence* is used when the incontinence is due primarily to underlying health problems rather than a mechanical problem within the urinary system. For example, even when the urinary system is functioning reasonably well, physical and/or cognitive disabilities such as immobility, severe arthritis, and Alzheimer's disease can make

Chronic Incontinence		
TYPE	CAUSE	SYMPTOMS
Stress incontinence	Increase in abdominal pressure causes loss of urethral pressure	Leakage with cough, sneeze, laugh, exercise, lifting
Urge urinary incontinence/ overactive bladder	Involuntary bladder contraction	Urgency, frequency, frequent night urination, urine loss with sudden urge
Mixed incontinence	Combination of stress urinary incontinence (SUI) and urge urinary incontinence (UUI)	Urine loss with all of the above, although one type may predominate
Overflow urinary incontinence	Urethral obstruction or weak bladder contraction—incomplete bladder emptying	Difficulty beginning urination, weak stream, dribbling, leaking
Functional urinary incontinence	Physical or cognitive barriers to toileting	Inability to recognize signal to go, limited mobility or dexterity

it difficult to reach the bathroom in time or to even recognize the signals that it is time to go.

Risk Factors for Developing Urinary Incontinence

So who develops UI, and why? Epidemiologists have been asking this very question for years.

Studies of the prevalence and risk factors associated with a given health problem require the long-term follow-up of large groups of people. Jeanette Brown, M.D., and her associates studied a group of 7,949 women who were enrolled in the Study of Osteoporotic Fractures (SOF). Participants in this trial were recruited from four different geographic areas in the United States and were between the ages of 69 and 101, living at home, and able to walk without assistance. All women received regular clinic visits over many years. They got physical examinations and were asked about their medical and surgical histories as well as the medications they took regularly. In the sixth year of the study, they were also asked

Factors Associated with Daily UI	Rate of Increased Risk
Oral estrogen use	90%
Stroke	80%
Diabetes	70%
Poor overall health	60%
Obesity	50%
Chronic obstructive pulmonary disease	40%
Hysterectomy	40%
Age over 65 (increases every 5 years)	30%
One or more live births	20–30%

about urinary incontinence. A little over 41 percent of the women reported UI at least once a month; 14 percent revealed that they had incontinence every day.[8] When the research group investigated the factors associated with daily UI, some of the results were surprising. Risk factors for developing UI are summarized in the table on page 224.

What can we do with this information? Identifying risk factors helps us to understand how UI may develop. And when we identify those health problems and behaviors that can influence our risk of UI, we can develop strategies for preventing the problem in the long term. Let's take the example of obesity. While we don't understand the exact mechanisms by which increased BMI (body mass index, a measure of normal versus excess body weight) contributes to UI, we can theorize that increased weight creates increased pressure on the bladder, intensifying the challenge to the urethra to stay closed. Excess fat may damage bladder support or impair blood flow or the nerve supply to the bladder. Are these changes reversible? Can weight loss prevent or improve incontinence? Studies conducted by researchers at University of California, San Francisco (UCSF), suggest that weight loss can be an effective treatment for incontinence. In one trial, incontinent women who weighed more than 200 pounds were enrolled in a weight-loss program. At the end of the program, it was shown that a 15 percent or greater weight loss (30 pounds or more in this group) resulted in a 50 percent or more improvement in UI.[9]

And what about the other risk factors listed in this chapter? We have some control over some, while over others we do not. Aging affects us all. None of us can stop the advance of time. Few of us would choose to forgo having children simply because of increased risk of developing UI later in life (and remaining childless is no guarantee of future continence). But knowing the risk factors for UI may increase your resolve to adopt health habits that lower risk for diabetes (weight loss, exercise, diet modifications), and women at risk for stroke may be encouraged to control blood pressure and/or stop smoking.

Diagnosing Urinary Incontinence

The first step in overcoming UI is seeking treatment. If you *think* you have a problem with UI, you are probably right. Many women feel embarrassed admitting that they have a bladder problem. Only babies can't control their urine, right? Wrong. And incontinence is not a normal part of aging, any more than developing high blood pressure is a normal part of aging. It may be common, but it is *not* normal. It is a medical condition. And it *is* treatable.

But UI is hard to talk about. We don't talk about UI with our friends and our families, and we certainly don't want to discuss it with our health-care providers. Understanding that UI is a health-care condition that it is common and treatable will help break down barriers to seeking help. There is no need to suffer in silence.

Now that you've decided to do something about UI, how do you begin? Talking with your primary health-care provider or gynecologist is a good first step. Often, complicated testing is not needed for making a diagnosis, and many treatment options have few or no side effects. Your family practitioner or gynecologist may be the first and last step you need to take in addressing the problem of UI. However, if you are considering surgery for your problem, or if previous attempts at treatment were unsuccessful, you may be referred to a urologist or urogynecologist (a gynecologist who specializes in disorders of the urogenital tract). Or you may be referred to a continence center, a practice that specializes in disorders of bladder function. Here's what you can expect at your first visit with your primary-care doctor.

A FULL GENERAL AND MEDICAL HISTORY

Your health-care provider will ask about your general medical and surgical history. Report any pelvic or gynecologic surgeries you have had.

You will be asked about your bladder function. Questions may include:

- How often do you urinate?
- How many times a night do you awaken to use the bathroom?
- Do you ever wet the bed?
- Do you leak urine? How often?
- Under what circumstances do you leak—e.g., coughing, sneezing, laughing, lifting, or exercising? When you hear the sound of running water?
- Do you leak with intercourse?
- How long have you noticed a problem with bladder control?
- Do you use sanitary protection against leakage, such as using a panty liner, incontinence pad, or protective garment?

You may be asked to keep a urinary diary, a written record of your daily urination, leaking, and perhaps your daily fluid intake. You may simply want to jot down this information on a piece of paper, noting the time each of these events occurred, or you may be given a sheet or booklet in which to keep this record. A sample of the diary we use at the UCSF Women's Continence Center appears on pages 228–229.

INSTRUCTIONS FOR FILLING OUT
YOUR URINARY DIARY

1. In the first column, mark an (X) every time you urinated into the toilet.
2. In the second column, mark an (X) every time you accidentally leaked urine.
3. If an accident occurred, indicate in the third column the reason or circumstances surrounding the accident (e.g., "coughed," "bent over," "sudden urge").
4. Under "Fluid Type," describe the type you drank (coffee, tea, juice, etc.) and the amount (1 cup, 1 quart, etc.).
5. Circle the time you went to bed and the time you got up in the morning.

6. In the designated space below the diary, record the number and type of pads used.
7. Under Notes, write any additional information, such as type and dose of medication you are on for your urinary incontinence.

Many women find that urinary diaries are helpful in identifying situations or times of day when maintaining continence is the most difficult. A written record can help you monitor your progress. You need not keep a diary every day, but recording your information one to three times a week can be helpful.

PHYSICAL EXAMINATION

Your health-care provider will do a physical examination that should include a neurological exam (to make sure that the nerves serving the bladder are intact and functioning) and a pelvic exam (to look for signs of atrophy or prolapse). You will be asked to give a urine sample, and this will be tested for signs of infection. You may also have a test to check the

Time	Urinate in Toilet	Leaking Accident	Reason for Accident	Fluid Type	Fluid Amount
6:00 A.M.					
7:00 A.M.					
8:00 A.M.					
9:00 A.M.					
10:00 A.M.					
11:00 A.M.					
12 noon					
1:00 P.M.					

Time	Urinate in Toilet	Leaking Accident	Reason for Accident	Fluid Type	Fluid Amount
2:00 P.M.					
3:00 P.M.					
4:00 P.M.					
5:00 P.M.					
6:00 P.M.					
7:00 P.M.					
8:00 P.M.					
9:00 P.M.					
10:00 P.M.					
11:00 P.M.					
12 midnight					
1:00 A.M.					
2:00 A.M.					
3:00 A.M.					
4:00 A.M.					
5:00 A.M.					

Number and type of pads used in 24-hour period:
Notes:

amount of urine left in your bladder after urinating. This test is called a "postvoid residual" or PVR. A PVR is done to rule out urinary retention (the inability to adequately empty the bladder) as the underlying cause of incontinence. This test is done either by inserting a small catheter into the bladder and draining and measuring the remaining urine or by using ultrasound (a sonogram of the bladder) to check for fluid remaining in the bladder after urination.

OPTING FOR FURTHER TESTING

For certain patients more specialized and expensive ways of evaluating bladder function are available. Urodynamic profile testing (UDP) is the broad term for a series of tests: cystometrogram, urethral pressure profile (UPP), urine flowmetry, and cystoscopy. UDP testing is generally reserved for those patients who:

- Have complex bladder problems requiring additional clinical information.
- Have tried a variety of UI treatments without success.
- Have other medical problems making accurate diagnosis difficult.
- Plan to have surgery for UI.

HRT and Treating Urinary Incontinence

In the recent past, health-care providers would often suggest that women with UI consider taking hormone replacement therapy (HRT). However, early studies in which postmenopausal women were given oral hormone therapy for UI symptoms had inconsistent results.

And in 2001, researchers at the University of California, San Francisco (UCSF), published results of a study that caused health-care providers to rethink their recommendations about using HRT for UI. They included questions about urinary incontinence in the Heart and Estrogen/Progestin Replacement Study (HERS). The HERS trial was designed to evaluate the effect of HRT on heart disease, and the 2,763 women participating were randomized (assigned by chance) to take either Prempro (a tablet containing estrogen and progestin) or an identical placebo pill. The study was blinded so that neither the researchers nor the women knew which pill they were given—the actual medication or the fake look-alike. At the start of the study, 1,525 women reported that they had UI at least once a week. The women were followed for a little longer than four years on average, and by the end of the study, 39 percent of the women with UI who were taking the HRT said their UI was worse, as compared with only 27 percent of the placebo group. The researchers concluded that "daily oral estrogen plus progestin therapy was associated with worsening urinary incontinence in older postmenopausal women with weekly incontinence" and did not recommend HRT for the treatment of UI.[10]

Later studies have confirmed these findings. The Nurses' Health Study has been following more than 100,000 nurses around the United States since 1976. The nurses receive periodic questionnaires about changes in health, medications, diet, and exercise. In 1996, the researchers identified 39,436 women between the ages of fifty to seventy-five who did not have UI. These women were re-evaluated after four years for UI. Among the nurses using systemic HRT (oral estrogen or estrogen patch, oral estrogen plus progestin, or the two hormones by patch and/or mouth), the rate of incontinence was 34 to 68 percent higher than in the nurses who took no hormones. The authors of this study concluded that "postmenopausal hormone therapy appears to increase risk of developing urinary incontinence. This risk does not vary by route of administration, type of hormones, or dose taken."[11]

From these large, well-designed studies it is reasonable to assume that there is no role for systemic HRT (hormones taken by mouth or in patch form) in the treatment or prevention of UI. But what about vaginal estrogen, which is often given to offset vaginal dryness or pain with intercourse that can occur with menopause? Vaginal estrogen can be administered either as a cream that is inserted into the vagina using an applicator several nights a week or through a medicated ring that is worn in the vagina for up to three months. When used in this manner, very little estrogen is absorbed into the bloodstream, but the effect on tissues of the vagina can be profound. Vaginal estrogen increases tissues elasticity, moisture, and thickness and reduces or eliminates vaginal dryness, irritation, and pain with intercourse.

Clinical studies have not convincingly shown a role for vaginal estrogen in the treatment or prevention of UI. However, estrogen cream and the estrogen vaginal ring (Estring) have been shown to be helpful for postmenopausal women who suffer from chronic urinary tract infections.

Treating Urinary Incontinence Today

Here's the good news, however. Not only is urinary incontinence a treatable condition, but there are lots of treatment options. Each type of treatment has some advantages and disadvantages, and which you choose will likely depend on your lifestyle, likes and dislikes, and personal preferences. Choosing the right treatment for you may come down to trial and error or mix and match.

Current treatments for UI fall into several general categories as shown in the table on page 246.

BEHAVIORAL THERAPIES FOR TREATING UI

A behavioral therapy is a treatment that involves the active participation of the person seeking treatment. In other words, you must do something—adopt a new positive behavior (such as doing an exercise) or reduce or eliminate an old negative behavior (for example, drink less coffee). The table on page 246 summarizes the types of behavioral treatments that have been found effective in managing incontinence. We discuss each in detail below.

Dietary Changes

A common question asked by women with bladder problems is, Should I restrict the amount of fluids I consume? Women with UI often limit the amount of fluids they drink in an attempt to minimize the risk of leakage. This is not always a wise decision, because it can result in overly concentrated urine, which may make the bladder more sensitive to smaller volumes of urine. On the other hand, overhydration (drinking more than 2 liters a day) is likely to have the same effect—that is, cause you to urinate more frequently. Younger women can generally use thirst as an appropriate signal to hydrate, but as we age, the perception of thirst may be dulled or slowed and there is a risk of dehydration. An easy gauge of adequate fluid intake is the color of your urine. A simple check of the toilet bowl will tell you. Look for urine that is the color of lemon juice. This light-colored urine signals adequate fluid intake. Too dark? Drink more water.

Women who find themselves needing to urinate frequently at night should focus on drinking more during the day and limit or restrict fluids after 6:00 P.M. or so. Moreover, certain types of liquids and foods such as alcohol, caffeine, concentrated citrus juices, and spicy foods may irritate your bladder, causing you to urinate more often. Keeping a urinary diary can help you to identify which foods and beverages challenge your continence.

Maintaining good bowel habits also is important for managing UI. Constipation or an impacted bowel can increase bladder irritability or interfere with proper urination. Make sure you are getting enough dietary fiber from your food—it is as important for bladder health as it is for good health in general. The best sources of dietary fiber include whole grains, fruits, and vegetables.

Pelvic Muscle Exercises to Improve Bladder Control

Pelvic muscle exercises, also called Kegel (KAY-gull) exercises, strengthen the group of muscles called the pelvic floor muscles. These muscles contract and relax under your command to control the opening and closing of your bladder. When these muscles are weak, urine leakage or loss may result. But like other striated (voluntary) muscles in our body, pelvic floor muscles can be retrained and restrengthened. Numerous studies have verified that pelvic muscle exercises (PMEs) work for women with UI.[12]

Although most continence specialists agree that PMEs can strengthen pelvic floor muscles (see figure 39) and help women with UI, there is no consensus regarding the perfect way to do them. There are, however, several principles for exercising properly and safely.

Begin by locating the muscles to be exercised:

1. Squeeze the area of the rectum to tighten the anus as if trying not to pass gas. Feel the sensation of the muscles pulling inward and upward.

    or

2. Insert a finger in your vagina and contract the vaginal muscles. The squeeze you feel will confirm that you are exercising the correct muscles.

The following are some tips for doing pelvic muscle exercises:

-   Identify the correct set of muscles. Many women with weak pelvic floor muscles will squeeze abdominal muscles, buttock muscles, even thigh muscles in a mistaken attempt to cause a pelvic muscle contraction.
-   Contract the appropriate set of muscles and hold them for an appropriate amount of time. Begin by squeezing to a count of 3 and then relaxing to a count of 3. As muscle strength and endurance improve, increase the count to 5, or 7, or eventually 10. Do enough repetitions to encourage muscle hypertrophy (thickening). This requires about 15 muscle contractions (one set) two to three times a day.
-   Pay attention while you are exercising. PMEs are physical therapy for a dysfunctional set of muscles. Don't think you can do this at stop signs while driving. You would never attempt to rehab any other injured muscle while driving, and your pelvic floor muscles are no different! And be patient. As with any physical rehab, it takes time to see results.

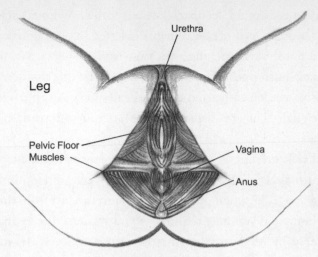

Figure 39: Pelvic Floor Muscles

- Give your program at least six to eight weeks for improvement
  to become apparent.

Set aside a short time each day for three exercise sessions. Choose times of day that are convenient so that you don't have an excuse not to do them—when you wake up, breakfast, lunch, dinner, and before bed are a few possible times of day.

Remember, this is a *muscle-conditioning exercise,* and like any other exercise, it is important to do it correctly in order to gain the most benefit. Focus on isolating the pelvic muscle and continue to breathe normally throughout each repetition. Muscles need oxygen to grow and strengthen.

Biofeedback

Biofeedback is a therapy that allows you to identify a physiological change within the body by a signal or number that tells you something about that change. For example, if you wear a pulse monitor while exercising, you receive information about how fast your heart is beating in response to increased activity. This is a form of biofeedback.

In continence care, biofeedback is used to help women identify and treat pelvic muscle dysfunction. Sensors inserted in the vagina or rectum or attached to the skin near the anus can detect the action of the pelvic floor muscles during pelvic muscle exercises. The information received by the sensors is then converted electronically into a graph, lights, and/or sound signals that are displayed on a computer screen and can be analyzed.

Biofeedback therapy is offered by many continence centers, urologists, and urogynecologists to help women learn and optimize their pelvic muscle rehabilitation programs. Sessions can last from thirty minutes to an hour, and you may require several sessions. Biofeedback therapy is covered by Medicare, but it is not always covered by individual medical insurers.

Weighted vaginal cones are a simple form of biofeedback. These tampon-shaped plastic devices are inserted into the vagina, and you hold them in place by contracting your pelvic muscle. Once you are able to hold a weighted cone in place for up to fifteen minutes, you move to the next higher weight cone.

Home electronic monitors are also available. Most are compact display monitors with a vaginally inserted sensor. Each contraction of the pelvic floor causes an electronic ladder or series of lights to escalate. These monitors can be helpful for women who have such severely impaired muscle function that they cannot feel their pelvic muscles contract. Visual or auditory feedback can indicate that the appropriate muscles *are* being contracted. Home units may not be covered by medical insurers.

Does using biofeedback make for better pelvic muscle rehabilitation? That depends. Some women find they can perform the exercises on their own with only simple instructions. But for women whose muscles are weak and functioning poorly, it may be difficult to feel the muscle contraction sufficiently to know whether you are doing the exercises correctly. For these women, biofeedback is a very useful tool in treating urinary incontinence.

Bladder Retraining

Bladder retraining is a well-established behavioral treatment for urinary incontinence that uses scheduled toileting to help you relearn normal bladder function. Bladder retraining can be used by women who suffer from either urge or stress incontinence.[13] The purpose of bladder retraining is to:

- Increase the amount of time between emptying your bladder.
- Increase the amount of fluids your bladder can hold.
- Diminish the sense of urgency and/or leakage associated with your problem.

Women are instructed to urinate at preset times during the daytime whether or not they feel the need to go. Schedules can be adapted individually, but it is important to stick to the schedule that you choose.

Start your schedule with intervals that are slightly challenging but achievable. For example, if you have been keeping a urinary diary, you might see that for three days in a row, you urinated every forty-five minutes to two hours. (It is important to keeping a diary of your bladder activity. This helps your practitioner determine the correct starting interval for you and to monitor your progress throughout your program.) Therefore, you might choose to begin your scheduled urinations at hourly intervals, beginning with the first morning void. Your subsequent urinations would occur hourly, whether you felt an urge prior to the hour interval or you reached the hour interval and felt little or no urge to urinate. The point is that you are reteaching your bladder that your brain is in charge of when to empty.

As you master this interval, usually in a week or so, extend the time by fifteen to thirty minutes until you achieve a normal voiding schedule—usually every three to four hours. If the pressure or urgency becomes difficult to bear, try a relaxation, distraction, or "urge suppression" technique.

BLADDER RETRAINING INSTRUCTIONS

1. Empty your bladder as soon as you get up in the morning. This begins your retraining schedule.

2. Wait the full amount of time before you urinate again, and when it is your scheduled time be sure to empty your bladder even if you feel no urge to urinate.

3. Follow the schedule during waking hours *only*. During the nighttime go to the bathroom only if you awaken and find it necessary.

4. When you feel the urge to urinate before the next designated time, use the urge suppression technique described below or try relaxation techniques like deep breathing.

5. Focus on relaxing all other muscles.

6. If possible, sit down until the sensation passes.

7. If the urge is suppressed, adhere to the schedule.

8. If you cannot suppress the urge, wait five minutes and then slowly make your way to the bathroom; then reestablish the schedule.

9. Repeat this process each time you feel an urge.

10. Your diary will help you see your progress and identify your problem times.

Urge Suppression

When a woman has a strong desire to urinate and is unable to reach a bathroom in time, this is called urge incontinence. The urge is a signal that it is time to urinate. Your goal is to maintain bladder control until you reach a toilet. A normally functioning bladder can wait until the appropriate opportunity to empty; an unstable bladder cannot. For a woman with urge incontinence, *rushing* to the bathroom when you have a strong urge to urinate is the worst thing you can do. Rushing actually causes increased bladder irritability and interferes with your ability to control your bladder. When urgency strikes, you should use the following urge suppression techniques to maintain control.

1. Stop all movement immediately and stand still.
2. Sit down if possible. Remaining still increases your ability to stay in control.
3. Squeeze your pelvic floor muscles quickly and tightly several times. Do not relax the muscles fully between these very quick squeezes. Squeezing your pelvic floor muscles this way signals the bladder to relax and increases your feeling of being in control.
4. Take a deep breath and relax.
5. Shrug your shoulders and let them go limp.
6. Release the tension in the rest of your body.
7. Concentrate on suppressing the urge feeling. Some women find distraction an effective technique.
8. When the strong urgency subsides, walk slowly and calmly to the bathroom.
9. If the urge begins to build again, repeat the above steps.
10. You can also try contracting your muscles as you walk to the bathroom.
11. Remember: Going to the bathroom is not an emergency!

ELECTRICAL STIMULATION

Because some women simply cannot identify or contract damaged or dysfunctional muscles, they may have trouble performing Kegel exercises or even biofeedback. In such cases, electrical pelvic muscle stimulation may be used. An electrical stimulation unit is a small battery-operated device (about the size of a TV remote) with a tamponlike sensor that is inserted into the vagina or rectum. When it is activated, it delivers a low-grade electrical current to create a reflex contraction and "unfreeze" stuck muscles. The devices usually have a switch that you can set for stress or urge incontinence. Electrical stimulation is usually used in combination with a pelvic rehabilitation program monitored by a continence specialist. Units must be ordered by prescription. Medicare may cover the expense of an electrical stimulation device if biofeedback has already been tried without success. Coverage by other medical insurers varies. Units can cost between $400 and $700.

SUPPORTIVE DEVICES FOR TREATING UI

Supportive devices are management aids for incontinence; that is, they do not treat the cause of incontinence, but using them can reduce or eliminate leakage. They can be used as a long-term option for managing leakage or as a part of an ongoing treatment program.

Pessaries

The pessary is a silicon rubber device that is placed into the vagina and worn like a diaphragm to support the uterus and/or bladder and rectum (see figure 40). While there are many types and shapes, the most commonly used pessary is a firm ring that presses against the wall of the vagina and urethra to help decrease leakage and support a prolapsed vagina or uterus (see figure 41). A pessary must be fit by a health-care provider. It can be worn daily or only when engaging in high-impact activities, and it can be removed nightly or even weekly and removed for

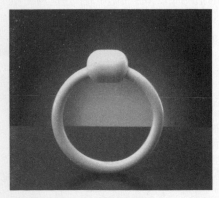

Figure 40: Pessary

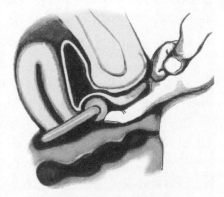

Figure 41: Pessary Inserted

periodic cleaning. A well-fit pessary should not cause any discomfort. However, not all women can be properly fit with a pessary. For those who can wear them, a pessary is an effective low-risk option for managing SUI.

Other Devices for Managing UI

There have been many attempts to develop over-the-counter and prescription products for managing UI. Patches worn over the urethra to block the loss of urine had a brief market life but were not widely used. Currently, a urethral insert called FemSoft is available by prescription. This fluid-filled sleeve is inserted into the urethra to block urine leakage. The urethral insert must be removed each time you urinate and replaced with a new device.

PHARMACOLOGICAL OPTIONS

Medications do not cure incontinence, but they can be very useful in reducing or eliminating problems of bladder control. Medications for the treatment of urge incontinence and overactive bladder, called anticholinergics, work by blocking unwanted bladder contractions. (SUI is caused by a loss of pressure in the urethra, and anticholinergics do not affect this condition.) Many of these drugs are safe for long-term use, although people who have glaucoma should check with their ophthalmologist before starting anticholinergic medication.

Currently there are no FDA-approved drugs for the treatment of SUI, but several drugs are in development. The table on page 242 lists some of the more commonly used medications for urge incontinence and overactive bladder.

Like many drugs, anticholinergic medications can have side effects. The most common side effect is dry mouth, which can range from mild to severe. Constipation and dry eyes are less common side effects. Rarely, drowsiness, confusion, or heart palpitations occur in people taking these

Pharmacological Options

Generic Name	Brand Name	Dosage	How to Use
Oxybutynin	Ditropan	5 mg tablets	½–2 tablets two to four times a day to a maximum of 20 mg/day
Long-acting oxybutynin	Ditropan XL	5–15 mg tablets	Once a day, up to 30 mg
Tolterodine tartrate	Detrol	1–2 mg capsules	2 mg twice a day, reduce to 1 mg if severe dry mouth
Long-acting tolterodine tartrate	Detrol LA	2–4 mg capsules	4 mg once a day, reduce to 2 mg if severe dry mouth
Oxybutynin transdermal	Oxytrol patch	3.9 mg/day 3" x 2" patch	Change twice weekly, every 3–4 days
Solifenacin succinate	VESIcare	5–10 mg tablets	Once a day
Darifenacin	Enablex	7.5–15 mg tablets	Once a day
Imipramine	Tofranil	10, 25, 50, 75, 100 mg tablets	10–100 mg once or twice a day
Hyoscyamine sulfate	Levsin	0.125 mg	1 tablet every 4 hours
	Levbid	0.375 mg	1 tablet twice a day

medicines. Depending on the specific medication, it may need to be taken once or several times a day to maintain effect. A patch form of oxybutynin is also available; it is worn on the abdomen, hip, or buttock and is changed every three to four days.

Prescription medications can be used alone or in combination with any of the behavioral treatments or support options discussed previously to manage UI. Sometimes it is a matter of trial and error finding the medication that will work best for you. Give a new prescription some time before deciding. I recommend a month's trial when trying a new medication.

SURGICAL OPTIONS

Surgery, in which the bladder neck and urethra are restored to their normal anatomical positions, is a treatment option for stress incontinence. There are three main surgical operations for urinary incontinence: bladder neck suspension, sling, and tension-free vaginal tape procedures—the last of which is a newer, less invasive procedure. The surgical approach used depends on a number of individual factors. If you are considering surgery, talk to your surgeon about which type of surgery is best for you. As with any surgery, be sure to choose a surgeon with a lot of experience specifically with incontinence surgery.

Bladder Neck Suspension

Bladder neck suspension is a procedure in which sutures (small stitches) are placed on either side of the urethra to create a cradle of threads that are anchored to strong ligaments or the pubic bone, providing support and stability. This procedure can be performed through the vagina with a long needle or through an incision in the stomach, and other pelvic problems (prolapsed organs, for example) can be corrected at the same time. Bladder neck suspension requires a brief hospital stay, though heavy lifting is generally prohibited for several months.

Sling Procedures

Pubovaginal sling procedures use a piece of strong connective tissue from another part of the body (typically from the abdomen) or from a cadaver to create a supporting hammock underneath the urethra and bladder neck to prevent leakage, especially during physical activity. It is becoming a popular procedure for treating UI because of its high overall success rate.

Tension-free Vaginal Tape (TVT)

Tension-free support is a minimally invasive procedure. Unlike the first two procedures, which are always done using general anesthesia, tension-free support can be performed under local anesthesia and takes only about half an hour to complete. Patients who undergo this surgery have a short recovery period and experience minimal scarring after surgery. TVT and similar procedures are relatively new, and it is not known whether the short-term success will last over time. However, the data so far is promising.

Periurethral Bulking Agents

Women who suffer from a form of SUI called "intrinsic sphincteric deficiency" (ISD) or "low pressure urethra" may benefit from bulking agents, which are injected at the junction of the urethra and the bladder base in order to cause the urethra to close. ISD generally causes leakage without an increase in abdominal pressure or an involuntary bladder contraction. The urethral musculature is simply weak and cannot maintain sufficient pressure to prevent leakage as the bladder fills. The procedure can be performed in the doctor's office or in an out-patient surgical center.

Currently, two agents are being used—Contigen and Durasphere. Treatment with either Contigen or Durasphere may temporarily interfere with normal urination, and women receiving periurethral injections usually are asked to remain in the medical setting until they have successfully voided. Only women with ISD benefit from periurethral injections, so it is important to be sure that you have been properly diagnosed before choosing this therapy.

SACRAL NEUROMODULATION THERAPY

Sacral neuromodulation (also called sacral nerve stimulation [SNS]) is a relatively new development in the treatment of severe OAB (see figure 42). InterStim, developed by Medtronics and approved by the FDA in 1997, uses a small device to send mild electrical pulses to the sacral nerve located in the lower back. The electrical stimulation may eliminate or reduce the bladder spasms causing OAB in people who have not responded to more conservative treatments.

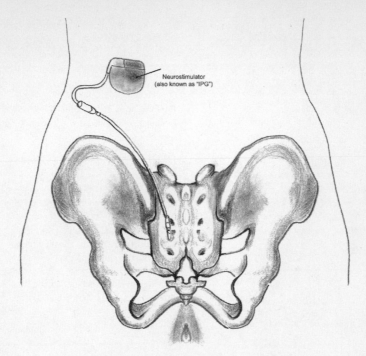

Figure 42: Sacral Nerve Stimulation (SNS) Device

During surgery, wires are threaded through open spaces in the pelvis and along the sacral nerves. The wires are then attached to a small electrical unit (neurostimulator) that delivers continuous electrical stimulation. The system is surgically placed under the skin (similar to a cardiac pacemaker) of the buttock or abdomen. Before the permanent device is placed, the patient is given a trial using an external unit. During this trial, the patient records her daily urinations and leakages in a diary for about a week. Then the unit is removed and the patient charts her daily urinations. If there is sufficient improvement, the permanent device is implanted.

Current UI Treatments	
CATEGORIES	EXAMPLES
Behavioral	Diet changes, pelvic muscle exercises, biofeedback, bladder retraining, urge suppression
Electrical stimulation	Liberty, Athena
Supportive devices	Pessaries, FemSoft
Pharmacological	Medications including Ditropan, Ditropan XL, Detrol, Detrol LA, Oxytrol patch, VESIcare, Enablex, Iofranil, Levsin, Levbid
Surgical	Bladder neck suspension, sling procedures, TVT, Contigen, Durasphere
Sacral neuromodulation therapy	InterStim

New Developments in UI Treatment

Researchers in Europe and the United States are reporting exciting new developments in the treatment of OAB. One interesting and novel approach is the use of a toxin injection of botulinum (the generic name for Botox). Small amounts of the neurotoxin are injected into several areas of the bladder, reducing unwanted bladder contractions. Though not yet approved for this use in the United States, results of trials of Botox for OAB appear promising. Initial studies report reduced urination frequency and less or no leakage within a week of treatment. Injections may need to be repeated periodically—every six months or so—but there is some evidence to suggest that the effect of repeated injections is cumulative, and reports of side effects are low.

Other researchers are investigating the use of capsaicin (found in peppers) to treat OAB, or small doses of medication instilled directly into the bladder.

The good news about urinary incontinence is that with so many treatment options available, there is no need to suffer in silence. Though common, incontinence is not normal. But it is treatable. So speak up. Talk to your mother, your sister, your book club. But most especially talk to your health-care provider and get some help.

Notes

Chapter 2. Sixty Years of Hormone Replacement Therapy: Where Are We Now?

1. Feldman BM, Voda A, and Gronseth E. The prevalence of hot flash and associated variables among perimenopausal women. *Res Nurs Health* 1985; 8: 261–68.

2. Barrett-Connor E, and Grady D. Hormone replacement therapy, heart disease and other considerations. *Annu Rev Public Health* 1998; 19: 55–72; Grodstein E, Manson JE, Colditz GA, et al. A prospective, observational study of postmenopausal hormone therapy and primary prevention of cardiovascular disease. *Ann Intern Med* 2000; 133: 933–41.

3. Stamper MJ, Willet WC, Colditz GA, et al. A prospective study of postmenopausal estrogen therapy and coronary heart disease. *N Engl J Med* 1985; 313(17): 1044–49.

4. Grady D, Gebretsadik T, Kerlikowske K, et al. Hormone replacement therapy and endometrial cancer risk: A meta-analysis. *Obstet Gynecol* 1995; 85: 304–13.

5. http:www.wyeth.com/about/period4.asp.

6. The writing group for the PEPI trial. Effects of estrogen or estrogen/progestin regimens on heart disease risk factors in postmenopausal women. *JAMA* 1995; 273: 199–208.

7. Collaborative Group on Hormonal Factors in Breast Cancer. Breast cancer and hormone replacement therapy: Collaborative reanalysis of data from 51 epidemiological studies of 52,705 women with breast cancer and 108,411 women without breast cancer. *Lancet* 1997; 350: 1047–59.

8. Schairer C, Lubin J, Troisi R, et al. Menopausal estrogen and estrogen-progestin replacement therapy and breast cancer risk. *JAMA* 2000; 283(4): 485–91.

9. The Women's Health Initiative Steering Committee. Risks and benefits of estrogen plus progestin in healthy postmenopausal women. *JAMA.* 2002; 288(3): 321–33; Shumaker SA, Legault C, Rapp, et al. Estrogen plus progestin and the incidence of dementia and mild cognitive impairment in postmenopausal women. *JAMA* 2003; 289(20): 2651–62.

10. Hays J, Ockene JK, Brunner RL, et al. Effects of estrogen plus progestin on health-related quality of life. *N Engl J Med* 2003; 348(19): 1839–54.

11. The Women's Health Initiative Steering Committee. Effects of conjugated equine estrogen in postmenopausal women with hysterectomy. *JAMA* 2004; 291(14): 1701–12.

12. Grady D. Postmenopausal hormones-therapy for symptoms only. *N Engl J Med* 2003. May 8: 1835–37.

13. Ibid.

14. Chlebowski R, Hendrix SL, Langer RD, Stefanick M, Gass M, Lane D, Rodabough R, Gilligan MA, Cyr M, Thomson C, Khandekar J, Petrovitch H, and McTiernan A. Influence of estrogen plus progestin on breast cancer and mammography in healthy postmenopausal women: The women's health initiative randomized trial. *JAMA* 2003; 289: 3243–53.

15. Stearns V, Beebe KL, Iyengar M, and Dube E. Paroxetine-controlled release in the treatment of menopausal hot flashes: A randomized controlled trial. *JAMA* 2003 June 4; 289(21): 2827–34; Goldberg RM, Loprinzi CL, O'Fallon JR, Veeder MH, Miser AW, Mailliard JA, Michalak JC, Dose AM, Rowland KM Jr, and Burnham NL. Transdermal clonidine for ameliorating tamoxifen-induced hot flashes. *J Clin Oncol* 1994; 12(1): 155–58; Loprinzi CL, Sloan JA, Perez EA, Quella SK, Stella PJ, Mailliard JA, et al. Phase III evaluation of fluoxetine for treatment of hot flashes. *J Clin Oncol* 2002; 20(6): 1578–83; Loprinzi C, Kugler J, Sloan J, et al. Venlafaxine in management of hot flashes in survivors of breast cancer: A randomised controlled trial. *Lancet* 2000; 356: 2059–63; Pandya KJ, Raubertas RF, Flynn PJ, et al. Oral clonidine in postmenopausal patients with breast cancer experiencing tamoxifen-induced hot flashes: A University of Rochester Cancer Center Community Clinical Oncology Program study. *Ann Intern Med* 2000 May 16; 132(10): 788–93.

Chapter 3. Herbal Therapies: East Meets West

1. Mills, Simon, and Bone, Kerry. *Principles and Practice of Modern Phytotherapy—Modern Herbal Medicine* (London: Churchill Livingstone, 2000), 421.

2. Ibid., 40.

3. Duker EM, et al. Effects of extracts from *Cimicifuga racemosa* on gonadotropin release in menopausal women and ovariectomized rats. *Planta Medica* 1991; 57: 420–24.

4. Stoll W. Phytotherapeutikum beeinflusst atrophiphisches vaginalepithel: Doppel-blindversuch Cimicifuga vs. strogenpr parat ("Phytotherapy influences atrophic vaginal epithelium-doubleblind study—Cimicifuga vs. estrogenic substances"). *Therapeutikon* 1987; 1: 23–31; Warnecke G. Beeinflussung klimatkterischer Besch-werden durch ein Phytotherapeutikum: Erfolgreiche therapie mit Cimicifuga-Monoextrakt ("Influences of phytotherapy on menopausal syndrome: successful treatments with monextract of Cimicifuga"). *Medizinische Welt* 1985; 36: 871–74; Lehmann-Willenbrock E, and Riedel H. Klinische und endokrinologische Unter-suchengen zur Therapie ovarieller Ausfallserscheinungen nach Hysterektomie unter Belassung der Adnexe ("Clinical and endocrinological examinations concerning climacter symptoms following hysterectomy with remaining ovaries"). *Zentralbl Gynakol* 1988; 110: 611–18.

5. Jacobson JS, et al. Randomized trial of black cohosh for the treatment of hot flashes among women with a history of breast cancer. *Clin Oncol* 2001; 9(10): 2739–45.

6. Fugh-Berman A, and Awang D. Black cohosh. *Alternative Therapies in Women's Health* 2001; 3(11): 81–85.

7. Upton Roy, editor. Black cohosh rhizome. *American Herbal Pharmacopoeia and Therapeutic Compendium.* Santa Cruz, CA, 2001.

8. Fugh-Berman A. Herb-drug interactions. *Lancet* 2000; 355: 134–38.

9. Nestel PJ, Pomeroy S, Kay S, et al. Isoflavones from red clover improve systemic ar-terial compliance but not plasma lipids in menopausal women. *J Clin Endocrin Metab* 1999; 84(3): 895–98.

10. Tice JA, Ettinger B, Ensrud K, et al. Phytoestrogen supplements for the treatment of hot flashes: The Isoflavone Clover Extract (ICE) Study: A randomized controlled trial. *JAMA* 2003 July 9; 290(2): 207–14.

Chapter 4. Managing Menopause with Traditional Chinese Medicine

1. Rossouw JE, Anderson GL, Prentice RL, LaCroix AZ, Kooperberg C, Stefanick ML, et al. Risks and benefits of estrogen plus progestin in healthy postmenopausal women: Principal results from the Women's Health Initiative randomized con-trolled trial. *JAMA* 2002; 288(3): 321–33.

2. Shumaker SA, Legault C, Thal L, Wallace RB, Ockene JK, Hendrix SL, et al. Es-trogen plus progestin and the incidence of dementia and mile cognitive impairment in postmenopausal women: The Women's Health Initiative Memory Study: A ran-domized controlled trial. *JAMA* 2003; 289(20): 2651–62.

3. Women's Health Initiative Steering Committee. Effects of conjugated equine estrogen in postmenopausal women with hysterectomy: The Women's Health Initiative randomized controlled trial. *JAMA* 2004; 291: 1701–12.

Chapter 5. Phytoestrogens and Natural Hormones

1. Kuiper G, Carlsson B, Grandien K, et al. Comparison of the ligand binding specificity and transcript tissue distribution of estrogen receptors alpha and beta. *Endocrinology* 1997; 138: 863–70.
2. Messina M, and Loprinzi C. Soy for breast cancer survivors: A critical review of the literature. *J Nutr* 2001; 3095S–3108S.
3. Cassidy A, Gingham S, and Setchell K. Biological effects of a diet of soy protein rich in isoflavones on the menstrual cycle of premenopausal women. *Am J Clin Nutr* 1994; 60: 333–40.
4. Anderson J, Ambrose W, and Garner S. Orally dosed genistein from soy and prevention of cancellous bone loss in two ovariectomized rat models. *J Nutr* 1995; 125: 799S.
5. Anderson J, et al. *N Engl J Med* 1995; 333(5): 276–82.
6. Han K, Soares J, Haidar M, et al. Benefits of soy isoflavone therapeutic regimen on menopausal symptoms. *Am Coll Ob/Gyn* 2002; 99(3): 389–40.
7. Walter S, and Jensen H. The effect of treatment with oestradiol and oestriol on fasting serum cholesterol and triglyceride levels in postmenopausal women. *British J Obstet and Gyn* 1977; 84(11): 869–72.
8. Follingstad A. Estriol, the forgotten estrogen? *JAMA* 1978; 239: 29–30.
9. Lippman M, Monaco M, and Bolan G. Effects of estrone, estradiol, and estriol on hormone-responsive human breast cancer in long-term tissue culture. *Cancer Research* 1977; 37: 1901–07.
10. Lee J. *What Your Doctor May Not Tell You About Menopause* (New York: Warner Books, 1996).
11. Hirvonen E. Progestins. *Maturitas* 1996; 23: S13.
12. Adams M, Register T, Golden D, et al. Medroxyprogesterone acetate antagonizes inhibitory effects of conjugated equine estrogens on coronary artery atherosclerosis. *Art Thrombo Vascu Biol* 1997; 17: 217.
13. The Writing Group for the PEPI Trial. Effects of hormone replacement therapy on endometrial histology in postmenopausal women. The Postmenopausal Estrogen/Progestin Interventions (PEPI) Trial. *JAMA* 1996; 275(5): 370–75.
14. The Writing Group for the PEPI Trial. Effects of hormone therapy on bone mineral density. Results from the Postmenopausal Estrogen/Progestin Interventions (PEPI) Trial. *JAMA* 1996; 276(17): 1389–96.

15. The Writing Group for the PEPI Trial. Effects of estrogen or estrogen/progestin regimens on heart disease risk factors in postmenopausal women. The Postmenopausal Estrogen/Progestin Interventions (PEPI) Trial. *JAMA* 1995; 273(3): 199–208.

16. Prometrium (progesterone, USP) Capsules. Package Insert. Solvay Pharmaceuticals. 1998.

17. Dobay B, Balos R, and Willard N. Improved menopausal symptom relief with estrogen-androgen therapy. Presented at the Annual Conference of the North American Menopause Society; Sept 1996; Chicago, Ill.

18. Watts N, Notelovitz M, Timmons M, et al. Comparison of oral estrogens and estrogens plus androgen on bone mineral density, menopausal symptoms, and lipid-lipoprotein profiles in surgical menopause. *Obstet Gynecol* 1995; 85: 529–37.

19. Rako S. *The Hormone of Desire* (New York: Harmony Books, 1996).

Chapter 6. Osteoporosis Is Not an Inevitable Part of Aging

1. Dawson-Hughes B, Harris SS, Krall EA, and Dallal GE. Effect of withdrawal of calcium and vitamin D supplements on bone mass in elderly men and women. *Am J Clin Nut* 2000 Sept; 72(3): 745–50.

2. Sinaki M, Itoi E, Wahner HW, Wollan P, Gelzcer R, Mullan BP, Collins DA, and Hodgson SF. Stronger back muscles reduce the incidence of vertebral fractures: A prospective 10-year follow-up of postmenopausal women. *Bone* 2002; 30(6): 836–41.

Chapter 7. Yoga for Healthy Bones

1. Greendale Gail A., et al. Yoga for women with hyperkyphosis: Results of a pilot Study, *Am J Pub Health* 2002 Oct; 92: 1611–14.

2. Hopper JL, and Seeman E. The bone density of female twins discordant for tobacco use. *N Engl J Med* 1994 Feb 10; 330(6): 387–92.

3. Michelson D, Stratakis C, Hill L, Reynolds J, Galliven E, Chrousos G, Gold P. Bone mineral density in women with depression. *N Engl J Med* 1996 Oct 17; 335(16): 1176–81.

Chapter 8. Managing Incontinence and the Overactive Bladder

1. Wilson L, Brown JS, Shin GP, Luc KO, and Subak LL. Annual direct cost of urinary incontinence. *Obstet Gynecol* 2001 Sept; 98(3): 398–406.

2. Kinchen KS, Burgio K, Diokno AC, Fultz NH, Bump R, and Obenchain R. Factors associated with women's decisions to seek treatment for urinary incontinence. *J Women's Health* (Larchmt). 2003 Sept; 12(7): 687–98.

3. Brown JS, Subak LL, Gras J, Brown BA, Kuppermann M, and Posner SF. Urge incontinence: The patient's perspective. *J Women's Health* 1998 Dec; 7(10): 1263–69.

4. Brown JS, Vittinghoff E, Wyman JF, Stone KL, Nevitt MC, Ensrud KE, and Grady D. Urinary incontinence: Does it increase risk for falls and fractures? Study of Osteoporotic Fractures Research Group. *J Am Geriatr Soc* 2000; 48(7): 721–25.

5. Brown JS, McGhan WF, and Chokroverty S. Comorbidities associated with overactive bladder. *Am J Manag Care* 2000 July; 6(11 Suppl): S574–79. Review.

6. Hunskaar S, Arnold EP, and Burgio, K. Epidemiology and natural history of urinary incontinence. *Int Urogynecol Journal* 2000; 11: 301–19.

7. Brown JS. Epidemiology and changing demographics of overactive bladder: A focus on the postmenopausal woman. *Geriatrics* 2002 May; 57 Suppl 1: 6–12.

8. Brown JS, Seeley DG, Fong J, Black DM, Ensrud KE, and Grady D. Urinary incontinence in older women: Who is at risk? Study of Osteoporotic Fractures Research Group. *Obstet Gynecol* 1996; May; 87(5 Pt 1): 715–21.

9. Subak LL, Johnson C, Whitcomb E, Boban D, Saxton J, and Brown JS. Does weight loss improve incontinence in moderately obese women? *Int Urogynecol J Pelvic Floor Dysfunct* 2002; 13(1): 40–43.

10. Grady D, Brown JS, Vittinghoff E, Applegate W, Varner E, and Snyder T. HERS Research Group. Postmenopausal hormones and incontinence: The Heart and Estrogen/Progestin Replacement Study. *Obstet Gynecol* 2001; 97(1): 116–20.

11. Grodstein F, Lifford K, Resnick NM, and Curhan GC. Postmenopausal hormone therapy and risk of developing urinary incontinence. *Obstet Gynecol* 2004; 103(2): 254–60.

12. Bo K, Talseth T, and Holme I. Single blind, randomised controlled trial of pelvic floor exercises, electrical stimulation, vaginal cones, and no treatment in management of genuine stress incontinence in women. *BMJ* 1999 Feb 20; 318(7182): 487–93; McIntosh LJ, Frahm JD, Mallett VT, and Richardson DA. Pelvic floor rehabilitation in the treatment of incontinence. *J Reprod Med* 1993; 38(9): 662–66.

13. Fantl JA, Wyman JF, McClish DK, Harkins SW, Elswick RK, Taylor JR, and Hadley EC. Efficacy of bladder training in older women with urinary incontinence. *JAMA* 1991 Feb 6; 265(5): 609–13.

Resources

Marcee Harris

Videos

*Approaching the 14th Moon: Women
  and Health Professionals Discuss
  Menopause*
Elizabeth Sher
Fax: 510-527-1031
www.ivstudios.com

*Between Us: A First-Aid Kit for Your
  Heart & Soul*
Mary Katzke, Affinity Films
212-979-6269

*Conversations at the Edge: Healing
  and the Spirit*
Rachel Naomi Remen, M.D.
Commonweal (retreat center)
415-868-0970

*Focus on Healing Through Movement
  and Dance*
Sherry Lebed Davis
800-366-6038
www.mobilityltd.com
shsh@mobilityltd.com

Healing and the Mind, volumes 1–4
  The Mystery of Chi
  The Mind-Body Connection
  Healing from Within
  The Art of Healing
Bill Moyers
shopping.yahoo.com/video/

*Look Good . . . Feel Better Caring for
    Yourself Inside and Out*
CTFA Foundation
800-395-LOOK
lookgoodfeelbetter.org

Therapeutic Touch
Janet Quinn, R.N., Ph.D.
303-449-5790
janetquinn@aol.com

Yoga with Stephanie Foster
800-759-1294
http://www.touchstarpro.com/

JOURNALS AND NEWSLETTERS

*Advances: The Journal of Mind-Body
    Health*
advances@fetzer.org

*Alternative and Complementary
    Therapy*
Mary Ann Liebert, Inc., Publishers
914-838-3100
www.liebertpub.com

*Alternative Medicine Alert:
    A Clinician's Guide to Alternative
    Therapies*
American Health Consultants
3525 Piedmont Rd., Building 6,
    Ste. 400
Atlanta, GA 30305
800-688-2421; Fax: 800-284-3291
www.ahcpub.com
customerservice@ahcpub.com

*Alternative Therapies in Health
    and Medicine*
Subscription Department
P.O. Box 615
Holmes, PA 19043-0615
800-345-8112
www.alternative-therapies.com

Common Boundary
301-652-9495
connect@commonboundary.org

*David Sobel's and Robert Ornstein's
    Mind/Body Health Newsletter*
800-222-4745

Dr. Andrew Weil's Self Healing
P.O. Box 2061
Marion, OH 43305-2061
800-523-3296 or 888-337-9345
www.drweilselfhealing.com

A Friend Indeed
Box 260
Pembina, ND 58271-0260
204-989-8028
www.afriendindeed.ca

Harvard Women's Health Watch
P.O. Box 420068
Palm Coast, FL 32142-0068
800-829-5921
www.med.harvard.edu

The Healing Arts Report
800-915-9335

The Healthy Mind, Healthy Body
  Handbook
David Sobel and Robert Ornstein—
  Center for Health Sciences
800-222-4745

HerbalGram
American Botanical Council
P.O. Box 144345
Austin, TX 78714-4345
800-373-7105
www.herbalgram.org

The Integrative Medicine Consult
P.O. Box 1603
Newburgh, NY 12551-1603
617-641-2300
www.onemedicine.com
consult@onemedicine.com

Nutrition Action Healthletter
Circulation Department
1875 Connecticut Ave. NW, Ste. 300
Washington, DC 20009-5728
Fax: 202-265-4954
www.cspinet.org/nah
circ@cspinet.org

The Soy Connection
Communique, Inc.
P.O. Box 237
Jefferson City, MO 65102
573-635-3265
www.talksoy.com

Spirituality and Health: The Soul/
  Body Connection
www.spiritualityhealth.com

Tufts University Health and Nutrition
  Letter
Subscription Department
P.O. Box 420912
Palm Coast, FL 32142-8242
800-274-7581
healthletter.tufts.edu

University of California, Berkeley
  Wellness Letter
Subscription Department
P.O. Box 420281
Palm Coast, FL 32142-0281
800-829-9170
garnet.berkeley.edu/~sph/Wellness
  Letter
well_ltr@uclink4.berkeley.edu

Yoga Journal
2054 University Ave
Berkeley, CA 94704
510-841-9200
http://www.yogajournal.com/

Recommended Books

Better Than Ever
Greg Anderson
New York: Harper, 1996

Breast Cancer: Beyond Convention
Mary Tagliaferri, Isaac Cohen, Debu
  Tripathy
New York: Atria Press, 2002

The Complete Book of Menopause
Carol Landau, Michele G. Lyn, and
  Anne W. Moulton
New York: Penguin Group, 1994

The Complete Woman's Herbal
Anne McIntyre
New York: Henry Holt, 1994

Dr. Susan Love's Hormone Book
Susan M. Love and Karen Lindsey
New York: Random House, 1997

Estrogen (3rd ed.)
Lila E. Nachtigall, M.D., and Joan
  Rattner Heilman
New York: HarperCollins, 2000

Estrogen: The Natural Way
Nina Shandler
New York: Villard Books, 1997

Healing Mind, Healthy Woman:
  Using the Mind-Body Connection
  to Manage Stress and Take Control
  of Your Life
Alice D. Domar, Ph.D.
New York: Dell Publishing, 1996

Herbal Healing for Women
Rosemary Gladstar
New York: Fireside, 1993

Listening to Your Hormones
Gillian Ford
Rocklin, CA: Prima Publishing, 1997

*Managing Menopause with Diet,
Vitamins and Herbs: An Essential
Guide for the Peri and Post
Menopausal Years*
Leslie Beck, R.D.
Toronto: Prentice-Hall Canada, 2000

Menopause
Isaac Schiff and Ann B. Parson
New York: Times Books, 1996

Menopause and Culture
Gabriella E. Berger
London: Pluto Press, 1999

*Menopause, Me and You: The Sound
of Women Pausing*
Ann M. Voda, R.N., Ph.D.
Binghampton, NY: Haworth Press, 1997

*Menopause, Naturally: Preparing for
the Second Half of Life*
Sadja Greenwood, M.D.
Volcano, CA: Volcano Press, 1996

*The Menopause Self-Help Book:
A Woman's Guide to Feeling
Wonderful for the Second Half of
Her Life* (4th ed.)
Susan M. Lark, M.D.
Berkeley: Celestial Arts, 1998

Natural Menopause
Susan Perry
Reading, MA: Perseus Books, 1997

*Off the Rag: Lesbians Writing on
Menopause*
Lee Lynch and Akia Woods (eds.)
Norwich, VT: New Victoria Publishers,
1996

Older and Wiser
Richard M. Restak
New York: Simon & Schuster, 1997

*On Women Turning 50: Celebrating
Mid-Life Discoveries*
Cathleen Rountree
New York: HarperCollins Publishers,
1993

Ourselves, Growing Older
Paula B. Doress-Worters
New York: Simon & Schuster, 1994

*Overcoming Incontinence:
A Straightforward Guide to Your
Options*
Mary Dierich and Felecio Froe
Indianapolis: Wiley, 2000

*The Pause: Positive Approaches to
Perimenopause and Menopause*
(2d ed.)
Lonnie Barbach, Ph.D.
New York: Penguin Group, 2000

Perimenopause
James E. Huston
Oakland, CA: New Harbinger
Publications, 1997

*Perimenopause: Preparing for the
Change* (2d ed.)
Nancy Lee Teaff, M.D., and Kim
Wright Wiley
Rocklin, CA: Prima Publishing, 1999

*The PMS & Perimenopause
Sourcebook*
Lori A. Futterman and John E. Jones
Los Angeles: Lowell House, 1998

*Reinventing Medicine: Beyond
Mind-Body to a New Era*
Larry Dossey
San Francisco: Harper, 1999

Screaming to Be Heard
Elizabeth Lee Vliet
New York: M. Evans and Co., 1995

The Silent Passage: Menopause
Gail Sheehy
New York: Pocket Books, 1993

*Staying Dry: A Practical Guide to
Bladder Control*
Kathryn Burgio, K. Lynette Pearce,
and Angelo Lucco
Baltimore: Johns Hopkins University
Press, 1989

Strong Women Eat Well
Miriam E. Nelson, Ph.D., and Judith
Knipe
New York: Putnam, 2000

Strong Women Stay Young
Miriam E. Nelson, Ph.D., and Sarah
Wernick
New York: Bantam Books, 2000

Strong Women, Strong Bones
Miriam E. Nelson, Ph.D., and Sarah
Wernick
New York: Putnam, 2000

Successful Aging
Anne C. Avery
New York: Ballantine Books, 1987

Transformation Through Menopause
Marian Van Eyk McCain
New York: Bergin & Garvey, 1991

Understanding Menopause
Janine O'Leary Cobb
New York: Penguin Group, 1998

*The Urinary Incontinence
Sourcebook*
Diane Kaschak Newman and
Mary K. Dzurinko
Los Angeles: Lowell House,
1999

*The Web That Has No Weaver:
Understanding Chinese Medicine*
Ted J. Kaptchuk
Chicago: NTC/Contemporary
Publishing, 2000

What Every Woman Needs to Know
About Menopause
Mary Jane Minkin and Carol V.
Wright
New Haven: Yale University Press,
1996

What Every Woman Should Know:
Staying Healthy After 40
Lila Nachtigall
New York: Warner Books, 1995

Women's Bodies, Women's Wisdom:
Creating Physical and Emotional
Health and Healing
Christiane Northrup
New York: Bantam Books, 1994

Women's Encyclopedia of Natural
Medicine: Alternative Therapies
and Integrative Medicine
Tori Hudson, N.D.
Los Angeles: Keats Publishing, 1999

COMPOUNDING PHARMACIES

Bellevue Pharmacy Solutions
1034 S. Brentwood Blvd.
St. Louis, MO 63117
314-727-8787

International Academy of
Compounding Pharmacists
P.O. Box 1365
Sugarland, TX 77487
713-933-8400

Lloyd Center Pharmacy
1302 Lloyd Center
Portland, OR 97232
1-800-358-8974

Women's International Pharmacy
12012 N. 111th Ave.
Youngstown, AZ 85363
1-800-330-0268

In addition, check your local
telephone directory.

LOCATING A PRACTITIONER, ACUPRESSURE

American Oriental Bodywork
Therapy Association
609-782-1616
www.healthy.net/aobta

LOCATING A PRACTITIONER, ACUPUNCTURE

American Academy of Medical Acupuncture
5820 Wilshire Blvd., Ste. 500
Los Angeles, CA 90036
800-521-2262

National Acupuncture and Oriental Medicine Alliance
253-851-6896
www.acuall.org

LOCATING A PRACTITIONER, BIOFEEDBACK

Association for Applied Psychophysiology and Biofeedback
303-422-8436
www.aapb.org

LOCATING A PRACTITIONER, HERBAL MEDICINE

American Holistic Medical Association
703-556-9245
www.holisticmedicine.org

Index of Herbalists
www.santabarbarahealth.net

LOCATING A PRACTITIONER, NATUROPATHY

American Association of Naturopathic Physicians
4435 Wisconsin Ave., NW
Washington, DC 20016
202-895-1392
www.naturopathic.org

Locating a Practitioner, Traditional Chinese Medicine

American Association of Oriental Medicine
433 Front St.
Catasauqua, PA 18032
610-433-2448
www.aaom.org

American Herbalists Guild
P.O. Box 70
Roosevelt, UT 84066
435-722-8434; fax 435-722-8452
www.americanherbalistsguild.com
ahgoffice@earthlink.net

American Holistic Medical Association
6728 Old McLean Village Drive
McLean, VA 22101-3906
703-556-9728; fax 703-556-8729
www.holisticmedicine.org

Herb Research Foundation
1007 Pearl St., Ste. 200
Boulder, CO 80302
800-748-2617 or 303-449-2265
www.herbs.org

National Acupuncture and Oriental Medicine Alliance
253-851-6896
www.acuall.org

General Women's Health Sites

American Medical Women's Association
www.amwa-doc.org

Centers for Disease Control and Prevention: Women's Health
www.cdc.gov/health/
womensmenu.htm

Health Finder
www.healthfinder.gov

National Council of Women's Organizations
http://www.womensorganizations.org/

National Library of Medicine
www.nlm.nih.gov/medlineplus/

National Women's Health Information Center
www.4woman.gov

Society for Women's Health Research
http://www.womens-health.org/

Wellness Web
www.wellweb.com

Menopause Organizations

American College of Obstetrics and Gynecologists Resource Center
P.O. Box 96920
409 12th St., SW
Washington, DC 20090-6920
www.acog.org

American Menopause Foundation
350 Fifth Ave., Ste. 2822
New York, NY 10118
212-714-2398
www.americanmenopause.org

The Hormone Foundation
4350 East-West Highway, Ste. 500
Bethesda, MD 20814
1-800-HORMONE
www.hormone.org

International Menopause Society
chez M. Steyaert
Av. des Cattleyas, 3, box 1
1150 Brussels, Belgium
www.imsociety.org
imsociety@Filink.net

Melpomene Institute
1010 University Ave.
St. Paul, MN 55104
651-642-1951; fax 651-642-1871
www.melpomene.org

Menopause Online
http://www.menopause-online.com/

National Women's Health Resource Center
120 Albany St., Ste. 820
New Brunswick, NJ 08901
877-986-9472
www.healthywomen.org

North American Menopause Society
5900 Landerbrook Dr., Ste. 195
Mayfield Heights, OH 44124
800-774-5342
www.menopause.org

National Centers of Excellence in Women's Health

The National Centers of Excellence in Women's Health were established by the Office on Women's Health in 1996. Their mandate is to establish and evaluate a new model health-care system that unites women's health research, medical training, clinical care, public health education, community outreach, and the promotion of women in academic medicine around a common mission—to improve the health status of diverse women across the life span.

Boston University Medical Center
720 Harrison Ave., Ste. 1108
Boston, MA 02118
617-638-8035
http://www.bmc.org/womenshealth/

Harvard University
Brigham and Women's Hospital
Neville House
10 Vining St., Room 202
Boston, MA 02115
800-417-4423
http://www.hmcnet.harvard.edu/coe/

Indiana University School of
  Medicine
Indiana Cancer Pavilion
535 Barnhill Dr., RT-150
Indianapolis, IN 46202
317-630-2243
http://www.iupui.edu/~womenhlt/

Magee-Women's Hospital
University of Pittsburgh
Department of Obstetrics, Gynecology
  and Reproductive Sciences
300 Halket St.
Pittsburgh, PA 15213-3180
412-641-4492
http://www.magee.edu/coe/
  homepage/home.htm

MCP Hahnemann University
  Institute for Women's Health
The Gatehouse
MCP Hospital
3300 Henry Ave.
Philadelphia, PA 19129
215-842-7041
http://www.mcphu.edu/institutes/
  iwh/iwh2/coe/coe.htm

Tulane and Xavier Universities of
  Lousiana
127 Elks Place, EP-7
New Orleans, LA 70112
1-877-588-5100
http://www.tulane.edu/~tuxcoe/
  NewWebsite/index.htm

University of California, Los Angeles
100 UCLA Medical Plaza Dr., Ste. 290
Los Angeles, CA 90095-7075
310-794-9039
http://womenshealth.med.ucla.edu/

University of California,
  San Francisco
Box 1694
2356 Sutter, First Floor
San Francisco, CA 94143-1694
415-353-2668
http://www.ucsf.edu/coe/

University of Illinois at Chicago
1640 West Roosevelt Rd., Room 503
UIC M/C 980
Chicago, IL 60608
312-413-3785
http://www.uic.edu/orgs/
  womenshealth/

University of Michigan Health System
Department of Obstetrics, Gynecology
1342 Taubman Center (Level One)
1500 E. Medical Center Dr.
Room L-4000
Ann Arbor, MI 48109-0276
734-936-8886
http://www.med.umich.edu/whp/

University of Pennsylvania
Center for Research on Women's
  Health and Reproduction
1355 BRB II/III
421 Curie Blvd.
Philadelphia, PA 19104-6142
http://www.med.upenn.edu/crrwh/
  cewh/

University of Puerto Rico
  Medical Sciences Campus
P.O. Box 365067
San Juan, PR 00936-5067
787-758-2525 ext. 1368

University of Washington
Women's Health Care Center
4245 Roosevelt Way, NE
Campus Box 354765
Seattle, WA 98105
206-598-7366
http://depts.washington.edu/uwcoe/

University of Wisconsin, Madison
Meriter Hospital—6 West
202 South Park St.
Madison, WI 53715
608-267-5566
http://www.womenshealth.wisc.edu/

NATIONAL CENTERS WITH HORMONE-THERAPY RELATED TOPICS

Alliance for Aging
2021 K St., NW, Ste. 305
Washington, DC 20006
202-293-2856

American Heart Association
National Center
7272 Greenville Ave.
Dallas, TX 75231
800-AHA-USA-1
http://www.americanheart.org

American Stroke Association
National Center
7272 Greenville Ave.
Dallas, TX 75231
800-4-STROKE
http://www.strokeassociation.org

Food and Drug Administration
Department of Health and Human
    Services
5600 Fishers Lane
Rockville, MD 20857
888-INFO-FDA
http://www.fda.gov

National Cancer Institute
National Institutes of Health
800-4-CANCER
http://www.nci.nih.gov

National Heart, Lung and Blood
    Institute
National Institutes of Health
NHLBI Health Information Center
P.O. Box 30105
Bethesda, MD 20824-30105
301-592-8573
http://www.nhlbi.nih.gov

National Institute of Arthritis and
    Musculoskeletal and Skin Diseases
National Institutes of Health
877-226-4267
http://www.niams.nih.gov

National Institute on Aging
National Institutes of Health
800-222-2225
http://www.nia.nih.gov

National Osteoporosis Foundation
1232 22nd St., NW
Washington, DC 20037-1292
202-223-2226
http://www.nof.org

National Women's Health Information
    Center
Department of Health and Human
    Services
8550 Arlington Blvd., Ste. 300
Fairfax, VA 22031
http://www.4women.gov

North American Menopause Society
P.O. Box 94527
Cleveland, OH 44101
440-442-7550
http://www.menopause.org

Office of Women's Health
Department of Health and Human
   Services
200 Independence Ave., SW,
   Room 730B
Washington, DC 20201
202-690-7650
http://www.4women.gov/owh

**Osteoporosis and Related Bone
   Diseases**
National Institutes of Health
800-624-BONE
http://www.osteo.org

National Centers for Urinary Incontinence

**American Foundation for Urological
   Disease (AFUD)**
3000 West Pratt St., Ste. 401
Baltimore, MD 21201
800-242-2283
http://www.afud.org/conditions/
   index. html

American Uro-Gynecologic Society
2025 M St., NW, Ste. 800
Washington, DC 20036
202-367-1167; fax 202-367-2167
http://www.augs.org

**National Association for Continence
   (NAFC)**
P.O. Box 8310
Spartanburg, SC 29305
800-BLADDER, 800-252-3337,
   864-579-7902
http://www.nafc.org

National Bladder Foundation
P.O. Box 1095
Ridgefield, CT 06877
877-BLADDER
http://www.bladder

National Institute of Diabetes and
  Digestive and Kidney Diseases
  (NIDDK)
3 Information Way
Bethesda, MD 20892-3580
800-891-5388
http://www.niddk.nih.gov/health/
  urolog/urolog.htm

National Kidney and Urological
  Diseases Information
  Clearinghouse (NKUDIC)
3 Information Way
Bethesda, MD 20892-3580
301-654-4415; fax 301-907-8906
http://www.niddk.nih.gov

Complementary and Alternative Medicine Organizations/Websites

ORGANIZATION	DESCRIPTION
Acupressure Institute 1533 Shattuck Ave Berkeley, CA 94709 800-442-2232 http://www.acupressure.com/ info@acupressure.com	The Acupressure Institute offers comprehensive vocational training in the areas of bodywork, Shiatsu, and acupressure massage. Website contains information about acupressure, healing books, instructional videos, charts, and tools for self-care.
Acupressure.org http://www.acupressure.org/	An informational website on acupressure definitions, origins, applications, books, and links.
HealthWorld Online http://www.healthy.net/clinic/ therapy/index.html	HealthWorld Online is a virtual health village with information, products, and services to help create a wellness-based lifestyle. Website covers information on natural therapies, diet, fitness, diseases, professional courses, and family health.
Alternative Health News Online www.altmedicine.com	Alternative, complementary, and preventive health news website offering information on wellness and natural approaches to staying healthy and living longer.
Alternative Medicine.com 1650 Tiburon Blvd Tiburon, CA 94920 800-515-4325 http://www.alternativemedicine.com	A website that integrates content from the organization's books, magazines, radio, and TV broadcasts to provide a comprehensive multimedia offering on alternative medicine health conditions, therapies, practitioners, and products.
The Alternative Medicine Foundation P.O. Box 60016 Potomac, MD 20859-0016 301-340-1960 www.amfoundation.org	The foundation provides consumers and professionals with responsible, evidence-based information on the integration of alternative and conventional medicine. Website contains databases of information, resource guides, and related events.

Complementary and Alternative Medicine Organizations/Websites

Organization	Description
Alternative Medicine Home Page www.pitt.edu/~cbw/altm.html	The Alternative Medicine Home Page is a jump station for sources of information on alternative, complementary, innovative, and integrative therapies. Created by the University of Pittsburgh, the site contains information on CAM literature, resources, and practitioners.
American Academy of Medical Acupuncture 4929 Wilshire Blvd, Ste 428 Los Angeles, CA 90010 323-937-5514 http://www.medicalacupuncture.org/	The American Academy of Medical Acupuncture promotes the integration of concepts from traditional and modern forms of acupuncture with Western medical training. Website contains patient education, provider referrals, a newsletter, and FAQs.
American Association of Oriental Medicine 433 Front St Catasauqua, PA 18032 888-500-7999 www.aaom.org	The AAOM is committed to enhancing the knowledge, competence, and expertise of holistic physicians to the greatest benefit of their patients. Web site contains complete information on the topic of Oriental medicine.
American Botanical Council P.O. Box 144345 Austin, TX 78714-4345 512-331-8868 www.herbalgram.org	The American Botanical Council is a non-profit educational and research organization disseminating science-based information that promotes the safe and effective use of medicinal plants and phytomedicines.
American Dietetic Association 216 W. Jackson Blvd Chicago IL 60606-6995 800-877-1600 www.eatright.org	ADA's mission is to promote optimal nutrition and well-being for all people through education and advocacy. Website contains information on lifestyle habits, policy activities, and a referral database of dieticians.
American Herbal Pharmacopoeia P.O. Box 5159 Santa Cruz, CA 95063 831-461-6318 www.herbal-ahp.org	American Herbal Pharmacopoeia disseminates information through quality-control standards for the manufacture of herbal supplements and botanical medicines focused on a high degree of safety and effectiveness.

(continued)

Complementary and Alternative Medicine Organizations/Websites

ORGANIZATION	DESCRIPTION
American Holistic Health Association P.O. Box 17400 Anaheim, CA 92817-7400 714-779-6152 www.ahha.org	AHHA promotes enhancing health and well-being through personal responsibility, considering the whole person, wellness-oriented lifestyle choices, and active participation in health decisions. Website offers informational articles, resource lists, and a referral database.
American Yoga Association P.O. Box 19986 Sarasota, FL 34276 941-927-4977 www.americanyogaassociation.org	The American Yoga Association is a non-profit educational organization that provides yoga instruction and educational resources. Website offers general yoga information, how to choose an instructor, and an online bookstore.
Arts and Healing Network ahn@artheals.org www.artheals.org	The Arts and Healing Network is dedicated to celebrating the connection between arts and healing. Website serves as an international resource for anyone interested in the healing potential of art.
Ask Dr. Weil www.askdrweil.com	Ask Dr. Weil provides online information and products for optimum health and wellness. Website contains information on a comprehensive array of wellness topics.
Association for Applied Psychophysiology and Biofeedback www.aapb.org	AAPB's mission is to advance the development, dissemination, and utilization of knowledge about applied psychophysiology and biofeedback to improve health and the quality of life through research, education, and practice.
Center for Mind-Body Medicine 5225 Connecticut Ave, NW, Ste 414 Washington, DC 20015 202-966-7338 http://www.cmbm.org/	A nonprofit, educational organization dedicated to reviving the spirit and transforming the practice of medicine. The center is working to create a more compassionate, open-minded, and effective model of health care and health education. Services include educational groups, professional training, conferences, and online resources.

Complementary and Alternative Medicine Organizations/Websites

ORGANIZATION	DESCRIPTION
Commonweal P.O. Box 316 Bolinas, CA 94924 415-868-0970 http://www.commonweal.org/	A center for service and research in health and human ecology. The program helps people seek physical, emotional, and spiritual healing.
Consumer Lab 333 Mamaroneck Ave White Plains, NY 10605 914-722-9149 www.consumerlab.com	ConsumerLab.com offers independent test results and information to help consumers and health-care professionals evaluate health, wellness, and nutrition products.
Fetzer Institute 9292 West KL Ave Kalamazoo, MI 49009 616-375-2000 http://www.fetzer.org/	The Fetzer Institute is a nonprofit, private-operating foundation that supports research, education, and service programs exploring the integral relationships among body, mind, and spirit. Programs include psychosocial effects on health, spirituality, and the relationship-centered care network.
Food and Drug Administration 5100 Paint Branch Parkway College Park, MD 20740-3835 800-322-0178 http://vm.cfsan.fda.gov/	The FDA, one of our nation's oldest consumer protection agencies, sees that the food we eat is safe and wholesome, the cosmetics we use won't hurt us, and the medicines and medical devices we use are safe and effective. Services include consumer advice, health information, and dietary supplement guidelines.
Herb Research Foundation 1007 Pearl St, Ste 200 Boulder, CO 80302 800-478-2617 www.herbs.org	The Herb Research Foundation is a reliable source of science-based information on the health benefits and safety of herbs—and in sustainable botanical resource development. HRF services include information searches, publications, a natural health-care hotline, as well as lectures and seminars.
Holistic Healthcare Online http://www.holistichealthcare.com/	A searchable directory for alternative health-care practitioners by state, country, city, or specialty.

(continued)

Complementary and Alternative Medicine Organizations/Websites

ORGANIZATION	DESCRIPTION
Holistic Medicine Resource Center 603-225-2110 mgold@holisticmed.com. http://holisticmed.com	A list of naturopathic Internet resources including national and international organizations, practitioners' database, Web-based discussion forums, and educational material.
Institute for Traditional Medicine 2017 SE Hawthorne Blvd Portland, OR 97214 503-233-4907 www.itmonline.org	An excellent resource for information on Chinese, Ayurvedic, Tibetan, and Native American medical practices.
Let's Talk Soy 800-TALKSOY www.talksoy.com	Let's Talk Soy is designed specifically for consumers, media, and the food industry. Consumer information includes ways to incorporate soy into a daily diet as well as facts and recipes for soy products.
National Acupuncture and Oriental Medicine Alliance 14637 Starr Rd SE Olalla, WA 98359 253-851-6896 http://acuall.org	The Acupuncture Alliance supports the development of acupuncture and Oriental medicine including a patient referral service of certified acupuncture and Oriental medicine practitioners, a quarterly newsletter, and advocacy outreach.
National Library of Medicine http://www.nlm.nih.gov/medlineplus/alternativemedicine.html	Alternative medicine page with current articles in alternative medicine and links to government resources.
National Women's Health Network 514 10th St NW, #400 Washington, DC 20004 202-347-1140 www.womenshealthnetwork.org	A national membership group that advocates for better federal health policies for women. Maintains a large array of information on a broad range of women's health topics. Newsletter available in English.

Complementary and Alternative Medicine Organizations/Websites

ORGANIZATION	DESCRIPTION
NIH National Center for Complementary and Alternative Medicine NCCAM Clearinghouse P.O. Box 7923 Gaithersburg, MD 20898 888-644-6226 http://nccam.nih.gov	NCCAM is dedicated to exploring complementary and alternative healing practices in the context of rigorous science, training CAM researchers, and disseminating authoritative information to the public and professionals. Website includes fact sheets, CAM databases, information on clinical trials, and links to federal government sites.
Nutrition.gov www.nutrition.gov	Nutrition.gov provides easy access to all online federal government information on nutrition. This national resource makes obtaining government information on nutrition, healthy eating, physical activity, and food safety easily accessible in one place for many Americans.
Office of Dietary Supplements National Institutes of Health 31 Center Dr, MSC 2086 Building 31, Room 1B29 Bethesda, MD 20892-2086 301-435-2920 http://dietary-supplements.info.nih.gov	The ODS supports research and disseminates research results in the area of dietary supplements. The ODS also provides advice to other federal agencies regarding research results related to dietary supplements.
Quackwatch www.quackwatch.com/index.html	Provides information to the public and professionals about hospice and palliative care. Services include a toll-free information and referral service, regional seminars, professional education, advice, and assistance.
Smith Farm Center for the Healing Arts 1229 Fifteenth St NW Washington, DC 20005 202-483-8601 http://www.smithfarm.com/	A nonprofit center for the study and teaching of healing practices, complementary to mainstream medicine that can lead to life-affirming changes.
Soy.com http://www.soy.com/	An online soy resource containing information, education, recipes, research, and other resources.

(continued)

Complementary and Alternative Medicine Organizations/Websites

ORGANIZATION	DESCRIPTION
Soyfoods Association of North America 1732 U St NW Washington, DC 20009 202-986-5600 www.soyfoods.org	The Soyfoods Association of North America is a nonprofit trade association promoting the consumption of soy foods. Services include health information, how to locate soy products, and current events.
Soy Information Clearinghouse http://www.soybean.org/	Excellent site for information on soy consumption including a soy foods guide, discussion forum, recipes, and newsletter.
U.S. Coalition for Natural Health www.naturalhealth.org	The mission of CNH is to protect every citizen's right to natural health freedom of choice. Website includes articles on various natural health topics, information on legislative activities, and a newsletter.
U.S. Soyfoods Directory www.soyfoods.com	Comprehensive website on all aspects of soy consumption and health benefits.
USDA Food and Nutrition Information Center Agricultural Research Service National Agricultural Library Room 105 10301 Baltimore Ave Beltsville, MD 20705-2351 301-504-5719 www.nal.usda.gov/fnic	FNIC's mission has been to collect and disseminate information about food and human nutrition. Site includes information on dietary supplements, guidelines, and links.
Yoga Journal www.yogajournal.com	A complete yoga resource with online information and bimonthly magazine.
Yoga Site http://www.yogasite.com/	A website with information on the various types of yoga, locating an instructor, links, and newsgroups.

Index